DUDE & DUDER

❖ HOW MY DOG SAVED MY LIFE ❖

Dude & Duder: How My Dog Saved My Life is published under Voyage, a sectionalized division under Di Angelo Publications, Inc.

VOYAGE

Voyage is an imprint of Di Angelo Publications
Copyright 2023.
All rights reserved.
Printed in the United States of America.

Di Angelo Publications
4265 San Felipe #1100
Houston, Texas 77027

Library of Congress
Dude & Duder: How My Dog Saved My Life
ISBN: 978-1-955690-56-0
Paperback

Words: Jeff Goodrich
Cover Design: Savina Deianova
Cover Photographs:
Interior Design: Kimberly James
Editors:

Downloadable via Kindle, NOOK, iBooks, and Google Play.

For educational, business, and bulk orders, contact sales@diangelopublications.com.

1. Body, Mind, & Spirit --- Inspiration and Personal Growth
2. Health & Fitness --- Men's Health
3. Self Help --- Personal Growth

DUDE & DUDER

HOW MY DOG SAVED MY LIFE

JEFF GOODRICH

To Duder, the best friend a guy could ever have.
To Holly (the Blonde), Daisy, and Roxie.
To my daughters, Talisha, Kairsti, and Dalayni.
To my grandkids, Lillyanah, Breeana, June, and Bear.
You are all my "why."

CONTENTS

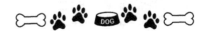

THIS IS MY STORY OF TRANSFORMATION

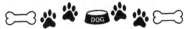

At forty-nine years old, my family and I adopted a Vizsla puppy. We named him Duder. This dog saved my life.

When I first asked my wife if I could get a dog, she reluctantly said yes, on some of the normal conditions of responsibility and such. I searched around and found a litter of puppies, made the arrangements, drove for a couple of hours, and picked up our little eight-week-old Vizsla.

Later that year, I turned fifty and went into a midlife crisis spiral of self-reflection and self-loathing. I was introspective to the point that I was living entirely inside my head instead of in the world around me. I was overweight, didn't feel content or happy in my own skin, and was always tired. My relationship with my wife was very rocky.

My job was so-so. All of my regrets about my life were top of mind. I wished I was a better husband. I wished I was a better father. I wished I was a better grandpa. I felt like I was just coasting along, day after day, just trying to survive.

Then along comes Duder, and he and I started going for a daily walk—sometimes around the neighborhood, sometimes on a hiking trail. These are the times that allowed me to truly ponder where my life was. But more importantly, it allowed me to ponder where my life needed to go.

From age fifty to fifty-one, I walked and talked with Duder every day. Three very important changes to my thought processes occurred during this year:

1. Awareness. I became conscious that I was unhappy, and I acknowledged this and accepted it.
2. Choice. I made a conscious decision to do stomething about it, to try and shift how I felt.
3. Why. I wrote down, studied, and pondered all the reasons why I needed to make changes.

When I turned fifty-one, I moved into the "do" state and went to work.

I am now fifty-five, and in the last four years:

- I have lost 70 lbs. and I am in the best physical shape of my life.
- I have run, and continue to compete in, half marathons, marathons, and ultramarathons.
- I learned to OWN all my choices. OWN all my

circumstances. OWN my side of relationships.

- My relationships with the Blonde, my kids, and my family have greatly improved and have recentered to be a core part of my life.
- The Blonde decided not to divorce me.
- My family adopted more dogs. Duder was our first, then Daisy (who is no longer with us), then Roxie. The Blonde and I currently have Duder and Roxie.
- I converted a van into a camper van, and the Blonde (my wife of 37 years), the dogs, and I go on adventures to fun and interesting places.
- My mindset changed to one of hope for the future.
- I wrote this book.

My life has transformed in virtually every aspect I can think of. And I am not done. I will continue to grow and live my life to the absolute fullest that I can.

Each chapter in this book represents a lesson that I have learned from Duder. These are all bits of wisdom that I have incorporated into my life.

I am Dude, my dog is Duder.

If change is needed in your life, then keep reading.

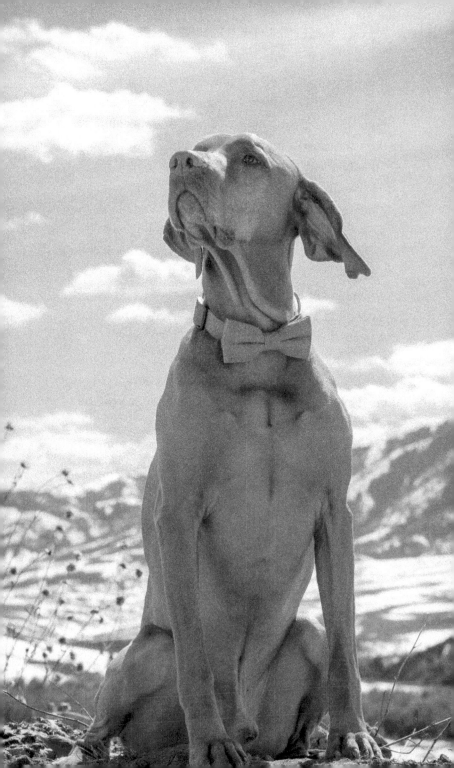

DUDER IS SPECIAL

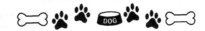

When I first met Duder, it was at a gas station where we picked him up. He looked at me, and the first thing he did was give me a lick on the face. From that moment, we became attached to each other.

He always wants to be with me. He follows me around the house and is always checking in on me. I believe he is making sure I am doing okay. If I am ever feeling anxious, he will walk up to me, put his head in my hands, and give me the attention and unconditional love that I need at that moment.

Duder became my therapist. I talk to him all the time. The act of speaking your thoughts out loud can be very beneficial, and he has always been willing to listen. He does not judge me, and no matter the circumstances, he is right there with me and by my side.

He is a very active dog and loves to run and play, all the time. This is inspiring and keeps me moving down this journey.

LIFE IS WHAT YOU MAKE IT

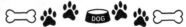

The basic premise of this book is a very simple one that has taken me many years to appreciate.

"Life is what you make it."

This concept applies to what you do, how you think, how you feel, how you respond, how you react, how you succeed, how you fail, how you process, how you treat others, and how you live and grow.

Every moment of every day, we make choices. Every choice we make defines who we are. A great line from the song "Freewill" by the group Rush sums this up: *"If you choose not to decide, you have still made a choice."*

A common theme I have heard from many inspiring people is to make choices for your future self. I had to truly get into the habit of considering the impact and fallout of my choices before making them. If I felt compelled to do something, I had to stop and ask if my future self would be happy about it. This simple idea had a big impact.

Life is what you make it, by the choices we make.

Every day is a new adventure, and Duder, Daisy, and Roxie have all taught me to truly appreciate this concept.

PUPPY TRAINING

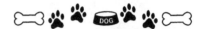

This is the first lesson I learned from Duder. Going through a puppy-training phase really inspired the idea of learning from Duder. What can this incredibly cute little puppy teach me, and how can I incorporate those lessons into my life?

When you begin puppy training, the first thing you work on probably has to do with the potty. Where is that dog going to pee and poop? How do I teach them not to go in the house?

Got me thinking...

I had made the choice to change my life, but where do I start? What is the first thing I should do? How do I do this? Who is going to help me? Do I need help?

Here are three things that had the biggest impact and served as starting points for me:

- I went for a walk, or a trail hike, every day with Duder. Duder needed that walk. He begged me to take him out. In my past, I spent a great deal of time sitting on the couch, watching TV and eating. Duder got me off the couch and out into the world.

- I cancelled my satellite TV subscription. If there was no TV to watch, then I could not sit down and watch it. I realized that the world TV portrays is not real. I needed to create my own world and my own reality.

- I started to read. I opened my mind up. I wanted to learn from others. I found books and podcasts that provided me with knowledge, ideas, and motivation.

From these simple things, my transformation had begun. I started to lose weight, my perspective was changing, and momentum was kicking in.

Everything starts with that first step. Take one.

DUDER HATES THE LEASH

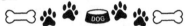

Most times, Duder has been able to go off leash when we hike. We are lucky to have a location that allows this. There are times when we need to put the leash on him depending on where we are. He hates it. He wants to run. He wants to go. He will look at me with desperation and anxiety, his eyes are saying, *Come on, Dude, why do I have to have this leash on? I want to run!!!*

Got me thinking...

When I hit fifty years old and began my life reflection exercise, I realized that for most of my life, I had put multiple leashes on myself. I was holding myself back. I was not allowing myself to run.

I can easily make excuses for this behavior. Blame my circumstances. Blame those people around me. It is easy to rationalize our bad behaviors that we know are not good for us. It is easy to hold ourselves back. Excuses, excuses, excuses. We use our backstory as our rationalization for our current choices.

When Duder is on that leash and we reach a location where I can unhook him, he launches full speed ahead, running in a full-on sprint.

There is no reason why we can't do the same. Once we learn how to take our leashes off, we can run at full sprint towards our goals. Make our dreams real. I like to visualize Duder taking off full speed down a trail. Pure happiness. I then equate this to me running towards my goals and dreams.

Don't let yourself down. Don't put that leash on. Unhook it. Let yourself go.

DUDER'S CHALLENGE

Write down what your personal leashes are.

The concept of our leashes is easy to understand. What might be hard is to truly identify what our leashes are, and then to flesh them out and understand them. This may take some time, but you need to take some time to truly document and figure out what they are. Once you do this, you can start to take action to take the leash off.

DUDER HAS A MISSION

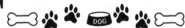

"That is what aggression is to me: The unstoppable fighting spirit.
The drive. The burning desire to achieve mission success using every
possible tool, asset, strategy, and tactic to bring about victory. It is
the will. To. Win."
—Jocko Willink

Duder is six years old now. We have spent a lot of time together, been to many places, and had lots of adventures. I am now convinced that he has a mission in his life. It is to be my best friend. All the daily routines and things he does all center around me and what I am doing, and he wants to be with me throughout it all. Duder came to us when he was a puppy, and he latched on to me very quickly. He has always wanted to make sure I am okay.

Got me thinking...

What is my mission? Do I have one? Do I need one?

When I began my transformation journey, the first podcast I ever listened to was by Jocko Willink. My daughter recommended it to me, and my first response was, *What is a podcast?* Well, since then, I've grown to become a great fan.

One theme Jocko emphasized in many of his episodes

is having a mission. He tied this into the military and that you always have a mission to complete. Many of our veterans come home from their service and have some hard times, sometimes because they do not have a mission that keeps them moving forward.

I have learned that having a personal mission is critical to your life in so many ways. It gives you hope. It provides you with goals to work towards, happiness and satisfaction, and something in your gut that drives you forward.

Looking back at my life before I turned fifty, I went through a period of about fifteen to twenty years of not having much of a mission in my life. On the surface, all seemed well. I had a job, had a wife, had a place to live, kids, grandkids. But I was coasting, doing just enough to get by. Not sure what my place in the world was, I was letting everything and everyone around me dictate how I was supposed to feel and what I was supposed to do.

I hit fifty years old and decided something had to change. I made a conscious choice. I can look back at the process now and describe it this way.

My first mission was to do different things than what I was doing at the time. That was it. Do something different. I wasn't even sure what or where to start, but I had a mission: Do something different.

I then took some time and made a list of what my mission in life could be, and more importantly, what it *should* be. This idea has grown and expanded over the last few years. I now have several very specific missions that I want to complete:

Mission #1 is to be the best husband, father, and grandpa that I can be.

Mission #2 is to inspire anyone who is currently in a place that I used to be in. These are the people coasting along in life. They know that something needs to change, but they're not sure what to do or how to go about it. I want to share my story. I want them to see that there is hope, regardless of your age or circumstance.

Mission #3 is to promote the power of dogs in our world and all the goodness that they bring to us in so many ways. Bring awareness to charities and other organizations that work with dogs and other animals.

Mission #4 is to promote how we can help our veterans and first responders in our communities. These brave people sometimes need assistance, and dogs can be apart of the healing process.

My overall mission is to be the best person I can be. As a husband, a father, a grandpa, and a member of my community. I choose to be impactful and make a

DUDER'S CHALLENGE

Take some time and think about your mission. Write it down. If you don't have one, find one.

difference in all that I do.

Duder had a mission. I now have one too.

WHY?

"Change your thoughts and you change your world."
—Norman Vincent Peale

Duder is a Vizsla, and dogs of this breed have some vibrant and dynamic basic instincts. They are very capable hunting dogs and are sometimes called bird dogs. I have not hunted with Duder, but the instincts are still there. When he is excited, he runs and jumps. When he smells another animal, he will go into hunting mode and sniff it out. Sometimes he will "point" at the thing, just like a good bird dog should do.

These are instincts. He does not know why he does them, he just does them. He does not need to know the "why."

Got me thinking...

Unlike, Duder, I needed to fully understand and find my "why." A great example of this is when I made the choice to lose some weight. My weight loss journey did not start with exercise, and it did not start with diet—it started in my mind. I refer to this principle as the Three Ms: Mind, Meals, Move.

This principle can be applied to anything you want to do.

I have wanted to lose weight over the last fifteen years and have made attempts at it. I have even joined a gym a couple of times with the intent to go "every day!" But those attempts failed. I can look back and understand that my mind was not ready. I did not have the discipline to continue. I did not understand my "why."

This time around, it started with my "why." I did not run out and join a gym. I put in place some thoughts and decisions that impacted my ability to have the required discipline.

Here is how I began my weight loss journey:

I had a trigger: I turned fifty. I had the full-on stereotypical crises, but I became aware of my shortcomings through them. I knew I had to change.

I made a decision: "I am going to lose weight."

I set a goal: Lose seventy pounds. When I started, I weighed 235 lbs. at five-foot-eight. My initial goal was to get to 185 lbs. I created a bunch of sticky notes that said "185." I put them everywhere in my house so everywhere I went, I saw the goal. It was at the top of mind.

Then, the most important thing for me, I wrote down my "why." I spent a great amount of time and effort defining this. Why did I want to lose weight? Why did I want to feel better? Why did I want to live a longer life?

This was a key aspect for me. This allowed my mindset to develop so I had the motivation to keep going. As time went on and momentum kicked in, my "why" continued to evolve—and continues to evolve to this day.

These ideas worked well when I wanted to lose weight. They also applied to everything I wanted to accomplish. I had to define, think about, and write down my "why." The process of writing this book followed the same Three Ms principle. The idea of putting all of this together into a book was a great idea, but why would I want to do it? To help me stay motivated and consistently work towards my goal, I wrote tons of little notes to myself that defined my "why" for this project—I keep them in a folder now.

I also believe that there will always be a part of your "why" that you cannot explain or even write down. It resides in your gut and in your soul. I learned that we have an enteric nervous system (ENS) that is two thin layers of more than 100 million nerve cells lining much of your digestive system. I believe that these nerve cells contain and control some of your drive and your "why." There

DUDER'S CHALLENGE

What is your "why"? Is there something that you want to do? Is there anything that you want to change in your life? Why? Write your answers down. Keep them visible at all times.

have been times where I would try not to "overthink" things and let my gut keep me going forward.

THE DUDER HEAD TILT

Duder will be sitting there looking at me, and when I do something that confuses him, he will tilt his head to the side. I can make a simple movement, like raise my hand in the air, and his head will tilt and his ears will rise a little. It always cracks me up to see how he's putting in real effort to try and puzzle it out. He'll do the same reaction to a strange noise or when someone gives him a fake, nonsensical command. You can see the gears turning in his head as he tries to work it out.

I always wonder, what is he thinking?

Got me thinking…

This idea of the Three Ms is now a core part of my thinking. I try to apply it in most things I do. When Duder does his head tilt, it is like he is thinking about it first and then trying to decide what to do. It always reminds me that I should, too.

Mind, then Meals, then Move. Here is how to apply this to anything you want to do.

Mind: I believe that everything starts in your mind. Start the process of figuring out your "why."

- What is the trigger that you need to do something?
- Are you fully aware of what you want to do?
- Envision your milestones. What does the future look like?
- All of your discipline will come from your mind; you are what you think you are.

Meals: Your body and brain need proper fuel to function.

- You cannot perform at your best at anything if you are not fueling yourself to perform optimally.
- What you eat affects the ability of your brain to function.
- What you eat just makes you feel good or makes you feel bad, so find the right food and fuel that work best for you.
- It is about what you eat, how much you eat, and when you eat.
- You are what you eat.

Move: This is the "do" component. This is where you get to work. The tools and techniques you use fit here. Everyone will have different success with different techniques, so find the ones that work for you and

embrace them.
- Set goals.
- Make a plan.
- Find a team.
- Define milestones and time frames.
- Meditate.
- Exercise.
- Define your "I am" statements.
- What is your self-talk?
- What is your mantra?
- Learn from others.
- You are what you do.

This gives you some ideas on where to start with something new or how to make a specific change. Over time, this thought process will just be part of how you approach everything.

FINDING OUR OWN WAY

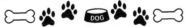

When we decided to get a dog, we already knew the breed we wanted. We found a litter of puppies and decided to go for it.

The day we picked Duder up was a wonderful one. From his perspective, though, it had to be tough. Here is a puppy, used to his mom and brothers and sisters. Then suddenly, he is taken away from them. He had to adjust. He had to learn about his new place in the world. New parents, new home, new food—all of it, new.

Got me thinking...

The Blonde and I have known each other since junior high school. We dated on and off during high school and were pretty much together for most of our senior year. At the end of our senior year, we discovered that she was pregnant. We were married three months after graduating high school. We moved into a small apartment together. We were two eighteen-year-old kids with a baby on the way, trying to find our way in the world. We were like

Duder, yanked from our normal environment to a new one almost instantaneously.

First thing was to figure out money and life direction. I had no idea what I was going to do. While working at our local pizza place, I decided to get a degree from ITT Technical Institute in Computer Aided Drafting. After graduation, the Boeing Company recruited me, and the Blonde and I and our first little girl, Talisha, packed up and moved to Seattle, Washington. This was the second time that we left all we knew behind and started again. We had no family out there. No friends. It was just the three of us trying to find our way.

When I look back on this experience, I can say that this was probably one of the best things we could have done. We were young and naïve, and we did not know the basics of surviving in our modern world. We were in a situation that required us to figure it out for ourselves.

While in Seattle, we had two more kids, and I finished a BS degree in computer science. We figured out how to live our life. We did it together. We learned together. We struggled together. We grew together. These early years of struggling were very impactful, and over time, those experiences have continuously helped us respond to life as it goes on.

Every one of us must find our own way in this world. As a parent, I have always wanted to make sure my kids were able to do the same. It is easy and natural to be that helicopter parent and give those kids anything and everything. The hard part of parenting is letting those kids make their own choices and let them celebrate or suffer through the consequences of their decisions and actions.

The Blonde and I have three different and unique daughters. Each of them has had their own successes and challenges in life. In the same way that I had to figure out my own path, my girls needed and need to do the same. Today, I see my primary role as an example to them. I want them to see me "doing" and "living" my life in a manner that inspires them. Ultimately, I want them to find peace and happiness.

ACCEPTING WHAT LIFE GIVES US

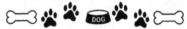

I am the oldest of five kids in my family. After I had moved out of my parents' house, at some point they ended up getting a dog. His name was Wiley.

When Wiley was around five or six, he started having seizures. My parents and siblings had to give him daily medications and care for him. Over time, his seizures got bad, to the point that he could not function, and my younger brother had to take him to the vet. At that point, they decided to let him go. Those were hard times.

Got me thinking...

When I was in high school, I started to have seizures. My personal seizure experience was not a pleasant one either. In the first draft of this book, I didn't even write about it. I have put those memories in the back of my mind as something that occurred in the past. I always tried to block them out and pretend they didn't happen. I didn't really talk or share too much about this with anyone. It was just something I, and only I, had to deal with. I guess I did not want to be labeled as an epileptic. I chose not to make it a part of who I was.

As I revisited some of these memories, I decided that there were some lessons to be learned, so I needed to write about it. These experiences played a significant role in my life, the Blonde's life, and our kids' lives. When I told them I was including this section in the book, my family shared things with me that I wasn't even aware of.

The seizures started in my high school days, and I dealt with the worst of them through my 20s and into my 30s. I have not had a seizure or a symptom of a seizure for many, many years now. I can't explain why they stopped, and I probably will never know. But what's equally bizarre is that the doctors could not find anything physical that would cause me to have seizures—no tumors in the brain or anything abnormal from MRIs or other tests.

If you haven't experienced a seizure, just imagine every muscle in your body actively contracting and relaxing as hard and as fast as they can. Every muscle. I was not awake for my seizures and cannot remember them, but I can remember the after affects. Every muscle was sore, like I had run a marathon as fast as I could while using every single muscle in my body. I would also have many sores in my mouth because my jaw muscles would contract, and I'd chew up the inside of my mouth. Sometimes I would have other injuries from falling or hitting structures or objects that were in my way during a seizure. For a couple of days after, my brain would be exhausted and not fully functional. I would have to sleep for long periods of time to recover.

After a few days, I would be on my recovery path, and I would feel fantastic for the next week or so. It could best be described as a brain reboot—like how your laptop always runs a little faster and better after a reboot. These were the times that I felt motivated, so I accomplished all kinds of stuff.

Many of my seizures would occur when I was sleeping, but they would sometimes happen in public places.

During the time when my seizures were at their worst, I was having a full tonic-clonic, or what used to be known as a grand mal, seizure every three or four weeks. They would be preceded by several smaller episodes, which are called "absence," or what used to be known as petit mal seizures. These were small periods of a very strange feeling; I can best describe it as extreme déjà vu. Part of my brain would just stop working. I could be having a conversation with someone, this unusual feeling would come over me, then I would just zone out. I would not have any idea what we were talking about or who the person I was talking to even was. At the same time, I still had the ability to walk away and go somewhere by myself until the feeling passed. I might've had a day where I had several petit mal episodes, and it would usually advance to a grand mal seizure. These seizures were hard on me, but for many reasons, they were just as hard—perhaps even harder on my wife and kids.

+

Back when we were in high school, the Blonde and I were out on a special date, and we went to a very nice French restaurant. I think I had an entire week's pay saved up to pay for this place. When we arrived and sat down, I had one of my petit mal seizures. Something was not right. I cannot remember the rest of the story, but the Blonde told me what happened. I had a petit mal seizure, so I got up and went to the bathroom. I went into a stall and had a grand mal seizure. I was just lying on the floor in the stall. After some time had passed, the Blonde knew something was wrong. She had to come into the men's room to check on me, and she found me lying on the ground. She crawled under the stall door and stayed with me until I was able to wake up enough so she could get me out of the stall. She got the money out of my wallet, paid for the food we'd had so far, then practically carried me to the car, and drove me home. I'm sure the people who witnessed all this just assumed that I was either drunk or on drugs.

+

Many years later, we were a young family in Seattle with three daughters. Our youngest was only a few weeks old and the middle one was about two. I was working for Boeing full-time and going to school at Seattle Pacific

University with a full load of credits. My oldest daughter, who was around seven or eight, had a soccer game that the two of us went to. After the game was over, we stayed and kicked the ball around. The field was empty by the time we started to head to the car. On the way, I fell to the ground and started having a seizure. No one was around, so my daughter had to run to another part of the park and find another game going on. She ran up to a coach and told him what was going on. He had to go find a pay phone to call 911. By the time the ambulance arrived, I was awake and becoming aware of my surroundings. I protested, but they still hauled me off to the hospital. This resulted in my driver's license being suspended. For the next year, I had to bike to work or ride with a coworker. And after work, I took two buses to get to the college campus for my evening classes. When my day was done, the Blonde would have to bring our kids with her in the car to pick me up at 11:00 p.m. because they were too young to be left alone, and the bus route didn't go near our house.

+

My youngest daughter recently shared with me that she never witnessed me having a seizure, but she remembers coming home from school one day and seeing me lying on the ground with the Blonde sitting next to me, petting my face and comforting me. She also remembers another time when she came to see me in bed after I'd had one, and she was startled by the blood on my shirt that came from my mouth. It scared her; she thought my chest was bleeding. For her, Dad having epilepsy was a weird and scary thing.

Sometimes she would think about it at night and become anxious, so she would open my bedroom door just to make sure I was still breathing.

+

In our bedroom in Seattle, we had a cedar chest against the wall opposite of the bed. There was a small walkway between the two. During one of my seizures, I fell down in this small walkway. This was a small and potentially dangerous place to have a seizure. The Blonde had to grab me, pick me up from that tight space, and set me down in an open area, all while I was shuddering uncontrollably.

+

My oldest daughter shared this memory with me:

She was at the house one day and I came home early from work. I was moving like a zombie and heading straight to my bedroom. At first, she only saw the right side of my face. But when I turned, she saw that the left side of my face was all beaten up and bruised. She ran outside to see if I had been in a car accident. Eventually, I was clear-headed enough to tell her that I had a seizure at work and hit my head on the toilet in the bathroom.

+

When I would have my petit mal seizures, I would often go into a trance or a zombie-like mode, as my eldest described. Sometimes I would even make some strange noises with my mouth, similar to smacking on food. To this day, the Blonde is triggered by this sound. Even now, when I am eating lazily and smacking my lips, the Blonde will whirl around to look at me, and then tell me to QUIT SMACKING!

+

I have been employed for several different companies and worked closely with many people in my line of work. Although I didn't want to talk about it, I knew my condition could affect others and that I should prepare them, so whenever I started a new job, I would tell the people I'd spend the most time with about my epilepsy. I would also tell them that if I did happen to have a seizure, they do not need to call 911. All they needed to do was make sure I keep breathing and that I have space. Luckily, I have only had a few incidents at my place of work. One time, I woke up on the ground in front of some elevators with a blanket on me. I don't even know how long I had laid there and how many people had to step by me to use the elevator.

+

These seizures became a part of who I was, but I still took a "whatever" attitude with them. Revisiting this aspect of my life has been an interesting exercise. The lesson is that everything that happens in our lives becomes part of who you are. These events shape you, and they also impact the people in your life. How we respond to these events is where we really decide who we want to become. We have to learn to accept what life gives us.

WHY DID WE GET A VIZSLA?

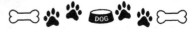

The American Kennel Club (AKC) recognizes 195 breeds of dogs in the world today, with many more breeds potentially being recognized. Out of all those options, why did we get a Vizsla?

Got me thinking...

Many years ago, before we had any dogs, the Blonde and I were hanging out at a friend's house. They had a Vizsla named Bear. As we were eating and chatting on the couch, this dog of theirs would not leave me alone. He gave me so much attention and followed me around wherever I went. It seemed like he wanted something from me. Turns out, I was wrong.

When we arrived, I was in one of my "pre-seizure" states. At one point in the evening, I had a petit mal episode, so I got up and went into the bathroom. I closed the door and had a grand mal seizure. Bear followed me to the bathroom, stood by the door, and started howling as an alert.

This dog knew from the moment I walked into the house that something was not right. He did not need anything from me—he was only worried about my wellbeing. He was keeping tabs on me, and he alerted everyone in the house when I had a seizure.

How did he know?

That's actually a very interesting question. Studies have been held on specially trained seizure dogs to understand how they can sense when someone is about to have a seizure. Some suggest that a person's scent, or pheromones, changes, perhaps via hormones in sweat or saliva. Others theorize that there are subtle changes in how someone moves, and some scientists even ponder if dogs can sense magnetic field shifts, as intense electrical activity occurs in the brain prior to such episodes.

But regardless of how, dogs are sensitive enough to humans that they can help. Trained seizure response dogs can alert their owners and others of an oncoming episode through barking or specific signaling. This can allow their owner to get to a safer space. If their owner is going to fall, the dog can put itself in between the person and the ground so it's not as hard as a landing. They can also be trained to push a medical alert button or alert the person that they may have a seizure coming.

This Vizsla named Bear most likely saved my life by alerting those in the house that I was having a seizure. That evening is when I decided that if I ever got a dog, I wanted to get a Vizsla.

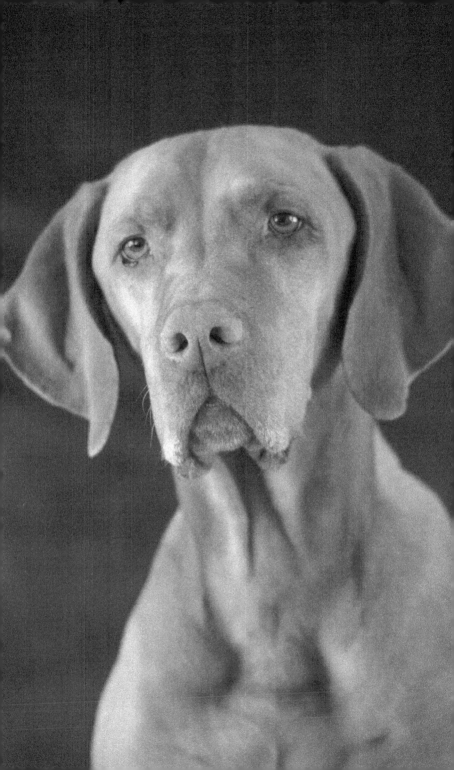

DUDER'S EARS

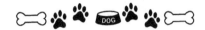

Duder communicates with me in many different ways. One way I like to observe is by his ears. Vizslas have some big and floppy ears. They do not stand up straight, but he does raise them. If he hears a noise, his ears raise and he gets alert. Sometimes in his more somber and quiet moods, they are simply hanging down the side of his head. It is a very relaxed state. I can usually get a feel for how he is feeling by looking at his ears.

Got me thinking...

When I hear the word "communication," my immediate thoughts are about the words I use and how I deliver them. But there is so much more to how we communicate. There are many books and information about this topic.

This really hit home with me when I discovered my alter ego. His name is Dude.

During the process of going through my

transformation, writing this book, and creating a brand, my alter ego was created. That is how "Dude and Duder" came about.

Dude became the guy that I wanted to be. He was the badass that ran ultramarathons. He was the guy that wrote this book. He was the guy that lost the weight. He was the guy that changed his eating habits. He was the guy that repaired his relationship. Dude was the man!

I often ask myself, "What would Dude do?"

When I would do this exercise and change myself into Dude, I noticed that I would naturally do some things differently. One simple thing that really surprised me is that I changed my posture. I put my shoulders back, straighten my back, and really put myself into a more confident stance. This made me realize how much of a difference the simple act of standing up straight can make. When someone looks at us when we are standing up straight, we naturally communicate confidence. This was huge for me!

I wish I could control my ears like Duder, though—his ears are awesome.

DUDER'S CHALLENGE

In our current world of sitting down all the time, standard posture has become a bit slumped. Check yours. Look up some exercises or techniques you could use to make it better, and practice them. Maybe, like me, you will see the impact it has on your confidence.

CLIMBING THE MOUNTAIN

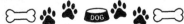

During my journey, I started an annual tradition. At least once a year, Duder and I would go on a backpacking trip together—just the two of us. Just a guy and his dog. These were great trips. Typically simple overnight trips, we'd go long distances with a pack on my back.

Backpacking is an awesome experience. The planning. Laying out all the gear you need. The process of minimizing it for weight management. Packing it in the small space of a backpack. The power in carrying everything you need on your back to survive for a couple of days. Spending that time and experience with an awesome companion named Duder.

Side Note: Have you ever slept in a mummy sleeping bag with a dog? I have.

One of the trips we took was to the highest peak in the state of Utah, King's Peak. This peak has an elevation of 13,528 feet and, depending on the route you use, it may entail twenty to twenty-five miles of hiking. This was not easy hiking, as there was lots of climbing, navigating big rocks, and some scrambling. We had to be diligent and cautious with the climb. As we were getting closer to the end, we had a view of the peak; we knew where we were going. We knew the challenge ahead of us.

When Duder and I reached the peak and looked out over the view, it was quite an experience. We stayed there for an hour, just soaking it in. Enjoying the moment. Talking with others that had made the journey as well. Then we started back down with a renewed feeling. The hard part was over. We met our goal.

Got me thinking...

As I started my transformation, I had many things change in my life: my mindset, my thought patterns, my self-talk, my relationships, my weight, my physical fitness, my perspective of life, my love for my family—all of it.

In the weight loss world, a very common event is that people would lose weight, then gain it all back at some point. There are many reasons and thoughts as to why this is. For me, I would have moments of my old self creeping back into to my world. This truly scared the hell out of me. I did not want to go back to my old self.

My transformation journey felt like I was climbing up King's Peak. I could see where I wanted to go. But I was not there yet. I had some hard climbing ahead. I was still going up. I felt like I could fall back down the mountain at any point in time. I could go back to my old habits and thoughts, back to my old patterns of eating and my laziness. Sometimes this is still a daily battle.

Overcoming old habits and old mindsets is hard. You truly must change. So, how do you keep climbing? At what point do you reach that peak and know you are over the top and you are the new you? These are questions that everyone must answer for themselves.

For me, I have not reached the peak yet. I am close, but I still have some more work and climbing to do.

Really got me thinking...

How was I going to make sure I did not retreat to my old comfort zone and bad habits? Two things worked for me. First, I had to embrace the idea that my transformation was a lifestyle change, not a temporary thing. Rather than being something I'd "try out" and "see where it goes," it would be a complete change in life. Second, I used the technique of doing one thing every day—my one thing that I had to do no matter what. I put all my mental energy into ensuring that I do that one thing every day without negotiation.

Running was that one thing for me.

I would go on a run every day. It didn't have to be a long one, but I just had to get outside and run every day. That became my anchor. I planted the seed in my head that I had to go for a run, and if I didn't do it, that was just plain unacceptable. It didn't matter the weather or the circumstance. I ran in the snow, in the rain, in the cold—you name it, I have run in it. When I travel, I schedule my runs into my travel plans. I plan my runs around races I sign up for. I plan my runs on whether or not Duder will be coming with me. I focused all my discipline on this one thing.

Here is my little disclaimer on this topic: There have been times where running is just impossible. I have had some injuries and illnesses that have prevented me from running for a week or so. But, when you do something every day, your body grows and adapts so you can continue that activity—it eventually becomes habitual. There will come a day when going on daily runs won't require the same amount of your focus and discipline, so your "one thing" will have to change. When running no longer works for me, I will just move onto something else that works—maybe biking.

What I found was that when you acknowledge your success with your daily anchor, then other things you want to do come a little easier. These are the daily successes that I take the time to acknowledge and give myself some internal kudos. This truly builds "grit" into your life and will expand to other aspects and areas of your life. Do that "one thing."

DUDER'S CHALLENGE

Find that one thing that you will do every day, NO MATTER WHAT. Make it your anchor. Make it your symbol of moving forward. Make it your symbol of discipline. Tell yourself, "If I do this, I can do anything else I want." This can be an action as simple as making your bed, going for a walk, doing yoga, meditating, or writing in your journal.

Find that one thing you can use to hold yourself accountable, do it every day, and use it to build needed momentum.

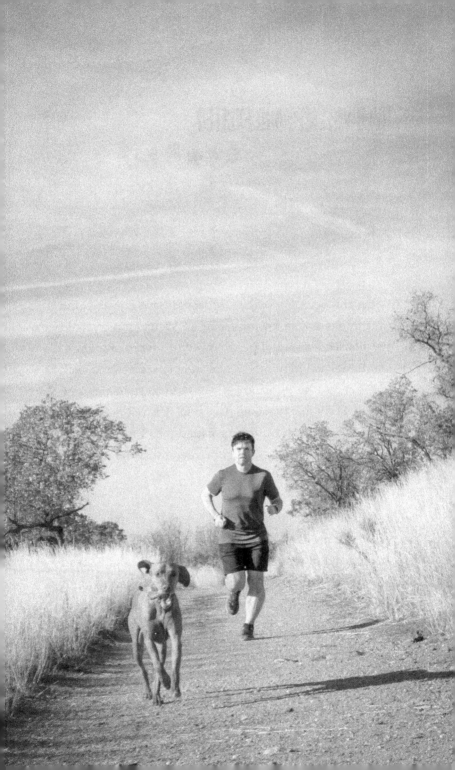

OVERWHELMED AND EXCITED

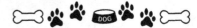

On the occasion where we would have guests come over to our house for dinner or an event, Duder would go nuts. This group of people would come in the house, and Duder would see them and want to say hello to each of them, but he didn't know where to start! Which one should I talk to? This one? This one? His tail is wagging almost to the point of being dangerous. He is running around the room, acting both very overwhelmed and excited.

Got me thinking...

When I hit fifty-one and started to change major aspects of my life, I sometimes felt like Duder.

I started to read books. But what book should I read next? There are so many to choose from! What type of book? Which are the best ones to try? Self-help? Finance? Personal development? Motivational? Science?

I started to listen to podcasts. Which one next? What type? Which ones will help me the most?

I started to work out and exercise, and I needed gear—so much gear. My social media feed filled with cool equipment that were all must haves! Do I join a gym? Which one? Should I do home workouts? Cross-fit? HIIT? Yoga? There are different types of yoga—what kind would be best for me? What's the best home equipment to get? Do I need home equipment? Do I need a heart tracker? A step tracker?

I started to run on a regular basis and needed to prepare for that. What shoes would be best? Do I need a water bottle? Backpack? Trail runs or road runs? How far should I go? How fast should I try to go? What is the best running technique? What should my cadence be? Should I sign up for races? When should I run? What should I eat? How do I track my running?

With all the books and podcasts, there were so many ideas coming into my head. Do I need to meditate—how long and when? Red light therapy? Blue light blockers? Cold showers? Cold immersion therapy? Should I practice self-talk? How do I develop a growth mindset and make choices based on my future self? How do I own my choices? When should I go to sleep? When should I get up? Do I need to journal? Start a gratitude practice? What does happiness look like for me? Should I track all my habits? Who should I follow on social media? Do I need that motivational calendar?

Do I need to change what I eat? What sort of diet should I go on? Keto? Intermittent fasting? Paleo? Vegan?

Pure calorie counting? Do I need a calorie tracker? Carb counter? How important is tracking what I eat? Tracking body fat? How do I even track my body fat? Will I need to take supplements? Which ones? How do I know what works and what doesn't?

I felt like Duder, running around with excitement over all this new information and these new possibilities. It was overwhelming, sometimes to the point of shutting me down. However, what I have realized over time is that my life is currently one big experiment. Everything I have done or tried has just added to my knowledge and experience, and this will still apply as I move further into my life. Getting excited and consuming everything there is to know about a new subject is my way of setting up for a new experiment; it's just preparing so I won't be overwhelmed when I dive in.

I have started to embrace the experimentation mindset. I am willing to try anything new—and that thing simply becomes an aspect of the journey. My journey is to experience new things.

Duder loves being excited, and so do I.

DUDER EATS GRASS

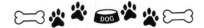

What the crap? It seems weird, but we will be out hiking or running on the trail, and he will stop and just eat the grass by the side of the trail. Why does he do this? Apparently, there are many ideas and opinions as to why he would do this, one of which is that he is not getting proper nutrition. Eating grass is a method to try and correct some nutritional deficiencies and digestive issues, so Duder is trying to eat better.

When we first brought Duder home, we did a lot of research on what to feed him and what his nutritional requirements were. I realized that I spent much more time researching what to feed him than what I should be feeding myself.

Got me thinking...

Mind, Meal, Move. While mindset is the most important aspect of weight loss, meal comes very closely after it. Nutrition is incredibly important. Our bodies require proper nutrition to function. How my body and mind function have a direct correlation to what I eat. This is not a radical idea.

During my weight loss phase of about six months, and then into maintenance mode, I have experimented with many different diets and eating patterns. I researched many different opinions and ideas from multiple people and nutritionists. I also started to log my food and was able to find correlation between what I ate, how I felt, and both my physical and mental performance. I also observed the Blonde, what she ate and how she responded.

My conclusion is that we are all different. We all have different requirements and needs for our maximum benefit. It took me some serious testing of food and supplements to find a good balance for me. Here are some of my findings:

What to Eat

Most of my weight was lost on the Keto/low carb diet. However, it was not just because of the low calories and low carbs that it worked. With my seizure disorder, Keto had a tremendous impact on my mind. It positively influenced how my brain functioned. When I am not on a low carb diet, I can feel it in my mind—I get what I call "brain fog," so I was not able to operate at my peak when I was eating a lot of carbs.

While the Keto diet was incredibly beneficial to me, it was not good for the Blonde. Her body and mind did not respond the same as mine. Keto is not for everyone. There are a hundred opinions out there about its effects, good and bad. It worked great for me for the pure weight loss mode I was in.

Simple things I do daily include: Avoid all types of sugars. Drink plenty of water. Get enough protein. Eat whole, non-GMO foods. Avoid processed foods. Listen to my body and respond to what it tells me.

When to Eat

I have incorporated basic patterns of when I eat. I practice some simple intermittent fasting ideas. I roughly follow a sixteen-by-eight plan: an eight-hour eating window and sixteen hours of fasting, only allowing myself to drink water. I will sometimes increase my fasting window when needed.

Supplements

I researched and tried out several different supplements designed to help me with what I was doing physically at the time. I currently do a lot of running, so I take natural supplements designed to help with things like joints, skeletal strength, and cardiovascular assistance. I do not overdo it. I take what I need.

Prescriptions

I am a firm believer in the power of our bodies' abilities to heal and operate on their own. The idea of the placebo effect is real, and I use it.

When I was first diagnosed with a seizure disorder,

the first thing the doctor did was run some brain scans. They did not find anything wrong, so the next logical step was to prescribe me medication. The first medication did not help or stop me from having a seizure, so they gave me a different one. This went on for about eight different types. It got to the point that the medication's side effects were worse than the seizures—and I don't even know if the medications I took had any long-term effects. I could not take them anymore. Things were much worse on the meds than off, so I eventually stopped taking them.

Looking back on this experience, I recall that none of my doctors ever asked me what I was eating as my normal diet. They didn't ask if I meditated, nor did they ask what exercise I was doing. They also did not recommend any changes in these areas. The answer was nothing but "try this drug."

This has given me a bit of a cynical view of today's basic medical method. It feels like the basic premise is that everything can be solved with a medication. Is this truly the best approach? I would say that most conditions people are diagnosed with can be tied to our eating and lifestyle choices.

Over the last three years, with significant changes in my mindset, my incorporation of meditation for my body's healing process, my eating habits, and my physical exercise, I have reached a point where I do not take any prescriptions. I also do not take anything that I consider manufactured. No aspirin, ibuprofen, Tylenol, etc. My body is operating on its own and operating how it is supposed to operate.

Another example is when I sprained my ankle while trail running. One run, I happened to step on a loose rock, and I twisted my ankle pretty bad as a result. When I got back home, it was swollen and sore. The normal "conventional" wisdom is to ice it and elevate it to reduce swelling and take something to relieve the pain. By this time, I had been living a much healthier lifestyle and my body was running efficiently, so I took a different approach. I did not ice it. I did not take any pain reliving meds. I let my body fix itself, as it is well equipped to do. I also brought my mind into the healing process. I was running again in four days.

In my experience, I have found my own body to be a master healer.

FEEDING TIME

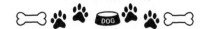

Duder loves to eat. He does get tired of the same old stuff we give him, so we try to vary it up a bit. Sometimes when we are eating, he will sit there and just wait. He is hoping for that small nugget of food that we might give him. He has also done his fair share of "counter surfing."

What I have observed is that he will eat most everything we offer to him. If he likes it, he will eat however much we give him. He will eat and eat and stuff himself if he likes the food.

Got me thinking...

I had always felt like I needed to eat everything that was put in front of me. If we went to a restaurant, many of which pride themselves on big portions, I had to eat everything on my plate.

What I realized is that we do not need to eat that much food. Our society has moved to this thought pattern of "bigger is better," which is not true. Understanding how much I ate as well as what I ate became important. I found that I could overindulge and eat too much, even if it was "good food," if I was not careful.

DUDER'S CHALLENGE

The three main things to focus on when establishing an eating pattern are: What do I eat? How much do I eat? And how often do I eat? Experiment with this. Research these ideas and find a pattern of eating that works for you.

DUDER IS AN OMNIVORE

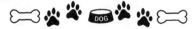

Duder will eat most things you put in front of him. He loves meat and he loves salad, especially if it has a good dressing on it. Based on that, he is what you call an omnivore.

So, what is his diet? We feed him a researched kibble and add additional meats and raw foods to the kibble. Am I supposed to call Duder an omnivore?

Got me thinking...

Making changes to your life includes changing your habits. One of the more impactful habits is what you eat. You are what you eat, and what you eat impacts every aspect of your life. Every. Single. Aspect.

The trick is to find the discipline to make the required changes and eat healthy. There are most likely things you are eating now that could be considered unhealthy.

What are techniques to use to get the discipline to stick to a diet? Here are some ideas I have learned.

First off, I hate the term "diet." It implies a temporary

time frame and temporary actions. There are times when you may want to do a juice cleanse, then you are on a juice diet for a defined period of time. However, what is your lifelong food intake going to be? Are you going to be on a "diet" for the rest of your life?

You need to make a choice. I choose to eat food that will have the best impact on my overall wellbeing, and I choose to avoid foods that will impact that bettered state. Once you have made that choice, then you need to find the foods that work for you.

Next, you need to change the way you think about it. For example, do you know any vegans? Notice the simple language. They are not on a vegan diet. They are vegan. Same with vegetarians; they are not on a vegetarian diet, they are vegetarian. This is who they are, and if they are that, then they will eat foods that fit that lifestyle. It is not a "diet."

For most of my life, I was eating what is referred to as the Standard American Diet (SAD). The SAD could be defined as an American pattern of eating consisting of ultra-processed foods, added sugars and corn syrups, and added fat and sodium. A lack of fruits and vegetables, whole grains, and lean proteins contribute to SAD as well. If most Americans eat this way and the majority of Americans are overweight and suffer from health conditions, it may be easy to draw the conclusion that diet plays a major role.

With experimentation, I believe I have found the types

of food that work for me. I have made the choice to make this my lifestyle and not a diet—instead, I made up my own term. I am "clean." Clean means natural, organic, non-GMO, and fresh. I have made my choice. I have made my statement. This is my lifestyle. I am not on a "clean" diet, I am clean.

DUDER'S CHALLENGE

Food intake is hard to change. Sorting through all the information out there is hard. Here are Duder's simple things to start with:

- Stop the soda and switch to water.

- Reduce and even stop the sugar, corn syrup, and glucose.

- Eat more fresh food and less processed food. If you take an inventory of all the food you eat in a day, how much of it would be consider processed?

  ⇨ There are different levels of processing from minimally to heavily processed. According to the United States Department of Agriculture (USDA), processed food is defined as any raw agricultural commodity that has been subject to washing, cleaning, milling, cutting, chopping, heating, pasteurizing, blanching, cooking, canning, freezing, drying, dehydrating, mixing, packaging, or other procedures that alter the food from its natural state. This may include the addition of other ingredients to the food, such as preservatives, flavors, nutrients, and other food additives or substances approved for use in food products, such as salt, sugars, and fats.

REWARDS AND PUNISHMENTS

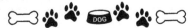

Duder gets rewarded for good behavior. Duder gets punished for bad behavior. This is a basic premise for training a dog.

Both rewards and punishments come in many forms.

Got me thinking...

When I was losing weight, there were many opinions, thoughts, and ideas that I read or listened to. One idea that has always troubled me is the idea of a "cheat day."

To this day, I have not fully resolved my support or disdain for this idea. I have been on both sides of the fence.

The idea of a cheat day is that you should take one day a week and eat whatever you want. The logic being that this is a reward for the diet or regime you have been on for the week. This idea planted a seed in my brain that when I would eat healthy, it was a punishment. When I ate whatever I wanted, it then became my reward. Isn't this backwards? Eating things that we know are unhealthy for us should be our punishment, and eating foods we know are good for us should be our reward.

During my transition, I had many little questions and mantras I would use and write on my whiteboard. One I liked was: "Are you going to do it or not?" So, every time I would be confronted with the delicious food that I knew was bad for me, I would ask myself that question. It helped keep me on track. So, are you going to lose the weight or not? Do you really need that cheat day?

One additional struggle I still have is, after running a race or a long run, I would have this thought that, okay, I just ran a race and had a good workout. I can "reward" myself with that burger, fries, onion rings, extra fry sauce, and large Dr. Pepper. Is this a good reward? Ask me the next day during my short run and I will tell you it is not.

I am still working on this. How do I define a reward versus a punishment? Maybe food should have nothing to do with rewards and punishment. Maybe my reward for a long run should be that new pair of running shoes! (I'm not sure the Blonde would go for that one though.)

But in all reality, the reward should and could be as simple as the internal kudos I give myself for that accomplishment.

At the same time, it changed what I considered rewards and punishments for Duder. A reward doesn't always have to be a treat. It can be a simple scratch of the butt. It can be a simple look in their eyes and smile. Dogs can feel and know when you are good to them. Punishment does not mean a scolding, or physical punishment. It can be a simple turning my back on him. He learns very quickly that maybe his behavior is not a good thing.

No matter what, he just wants his butt scratched.

DUDER AND THE MIRROR

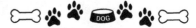

In our current living conditions, the Blonde has a mirror that is on the floor so she can practice yoga. The dogs can see themselves in this mirror when they walk by. When I first saw Duder look at himself in the mirror, he was very confused. He could see a dog in there, but he couldn't smell him—couldn't find its butt to sniff. It was like he couldn't process what he was looking at.

Does Duder know who he is?

Got me thinking...

I am going to describe two different people:

Person #1
- Happily married for over thirty-five years
- Has three awesome and loving daughters
- Has four awesome and loving grandkids
- Has a good job
- Owns a house
- Is physically healthy
- Enjoys life

<u>Person #2</u>

- Has had a rocky marriage and has come close to divorce many times
- Has experienced epileptic seizures for most his life
- Was laid off from two different jobs
- Had to file for bankruptcy
- Was a millionaire on paper, but it vanished over night
- Has a daughter who was a drug addict and saw life as a constant struggle

As you may have guessed, both of these people are me. When I look in the mirror, who do I see? Who do I identify as? In the past, it may have been #2. With some work on my mindset, I am now #1.

The point is that your identity and your life is what YOU tell yourself it is. It is not what others tell you, it is not what the world tells you, and it is not what your family may tell you. Do you want to live a negative life or a positive life?

There were times in my life that I felt like Duder, looking in the mirror and not knowing who I was looking at.

I have since found myself and I now know who the man in the mirror really is.

DUDER KNOWS ME

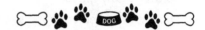

When Duder first came home to us, I was overweight. The bonding between a dog and owner occurred when I weighed 235 lbs. Soon after, I lost 70 lbs. I physically looked a little different, but Duder did not stop knowing me.

Got me thinking...

Who are we? Are we only defined by our outward appearance? What other aspects of me did Duder know? Was it my smell? Was it my voice? Was it my mannerisms?

What aspects of ourselves truly define who we are?

I think the first thing we should be worried about is who we are in our own minds. We spend a great deal more time interacting with ourselves than with anyone else. What are those conversations like?

In my past, when I was not in the place I wanted to be, I spent a great deal of time arguing with myself, being angry at myself. I realize now that most of my time with myself was mostly negative. I did not have a good relationship with me.

It took a great deal of time for me to adjust this pattern. The image I had of myself, I found, would be projected outward to those around me. It had an impact on every aspect of my life.

It was easy for me to try and point to external circumstances and blame them instead: It was the stress of the job. Someone said something to me I did not like. The Blonde was not exactly nice today. These are all things that would dictate my internal conversations. I was always looking for someone or something else to blame.

I learned to embrace the idea that I owned all my choices, they were all mine. This included how I felt, how I responded to people, and how I responded to situations.

One key thing that helped me a great deal was to truly understand that my life is mine. My life is what I was going to make it be. It was not going to defined by others or other situations. It wasn't that I did not care what others thought, I just did not live my life for them; I lived my life for me.

Over time, my internal conversations got better. I began to feel better about myself. I came to terms with me and who I was. Once I got here, I could then take the proper steps to grow and be a better person, and I eventually learned to like that person.

How this all got projected to those around me was fairly evident. Things did not bother me as much. I smiled more. I was more interested in others and what was going on in their lives than my own.

This was a critical step in my progress.

DUDER'S CHALLENGE

Take some time to evaluate your conversations with yourself. Do they need to change?

Here is an exercise you can try. Find a mirror. Look at yourself and talk to that person in the reflection. Ask yourself some fundamental questions, such as:

- Do I like myself?
- Do I feel like a victim of my circumstances and that there is nothing I can do about it?
- Is there any meaning in my life?
- What gives me hope?
- What can I do differently?
- How can I improve my mindset?

TAKING PICTURES, AND PICTURES, AND PICTURES...

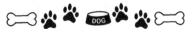

The Blonde maintains an Instagram page for our pups (@duderandroxie). She gets obsessed with taking pictures. Every place we go, every hike we take, every adventure we go on, she needs to get pics for the page.

Duder and Roxie have been trained for it now; they know that when Mom pulls out the camera and treats, they should probably just sit down and smile. It is inevitable and cannot be stopped.

There are times when it is frustrating for me. I just want to hike, but we stop every 100 feet because there is cool scenery or some cool flowers. So, we must stop. My role is the dog positioner. I drag the pups over the perfect place. Make them sit or lay down.

Got me thinking...

Many aspects of our lives can feel like they are out of our control, things that we just must do. We look at these things as chores, and they always have a negative aspect to them. We view them as stupid.

There are times when simply changing the way we look at these chores can make them a little more tolerable. Ask yourself: Why do I have to do this? What is the end goal? Is there a light at the end?

For the picture taking process, the end goal is a happy wife. So, ultimately, the end goal is happiness. This is a good result, so I always try to change my perspective and focus on that. There is a reason that I have to stop every 100 feet and take my role as dog positioner.

The dogs seem to get this. Their end goal is a delicious treat. So, they stop, they pose, they smile, and they try to make the Blonde happy too.

If you have something that you don't like to do, but it's something you have to do—there's no way out of it—you may have to change how you think about it.

Maybe the Blonde needs to bring some treats for me on the hikes.

VELCRO

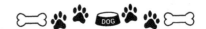

Vizsla's are known as Velcro dogs. Duder always has to be by my side and follow me around. He has to have me in sight. He loves to sit on my lap at every opportunity. And yes, he even sleeps with me.

He craves the physical contact. Over time, I got quite used to it. I wanted the same physical contact as well.

Got me thinking...

How does this relate to my relationship with the Blonde? She certainly craves and needs physical contact more than I do. I am talking about simple stuff. Holding her hand. Hugs, and lots of hugs. Sitting next to her when possible. Massaging her feet and back.

These simple acts of physical contact can have a tremendous impact on her emotional wellbeing. There are numerous studies and research that talk about the value and need for some of this simple physical contact. Duder taught me how important this is. I began to make a more conscious effort to have more physical contact with the Blonde after learning of its importance. It is amazing how this impacted our relationship!

NEW MEMBER OF THE FAMILY

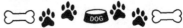

At some point in our dog owning experience, we decided to get Duder a little sister. Say hello to Daisy. She is a Vizsla, just like Duder. We were happy to give her a home and new big brother. We picked her out of a litter of pups and brought her home.

Got me thinking...

Neither Daisy nor Duder picked who their owners would be. They did not choose their family. This is true for us as well. We all have families, and we did not pick any of them. I chose the Blonde but did not choose her family, and vice versa.

Families can be fun and sometimes frustrating. But, like everything in life, how we respond to them and how we interact with them is on us. It is our choice whether to make it a bad or a good experience.

Duder and Daisy had to figure out how to get along with each other. They found a way. There are times when each of us have to figure out a way to get along with our families. If they are important to you, then you will find a way.

Duder and Daisy are happy with us. Let's learn from Duder; if someone from your family feeds you, be happy and lick their face. Or just make the best of any situation that may come up. Make a choice to make all of your family important to you.

ATTACHMENT AND HEARTBREAK

One day, the Blonde and I took Duder and Daisy out for a walk in the hills by our house. It is a good place to go since it has many trails and the dogs can run off their leashes. On our way back from the walk, Daisy was running along ahead of us, and she ran out into a dirt road and was hit by a truck. We did not see it happen, but we heard her cry out. We were scared. We ran to where she was, not knowing what we would find. She had made her way off the road and down into a small ditch. She was in pain and obviously very scared, and she seemed to be in shock. She had some serious injuries and one of her back legs was messed up.

The Blonde quickly called our vet. He was about to close shop for the day, but he agreed to stay there while we brought her in. I climbed down into the ditch and did my best to carefully pick her up. She did not know how to respond to what was happening to her. I was able to carry her to the truck, and I held onto her as the Blonde drove us to the vet.

The vet met us at the door and began some initial examinations. It did not look good. He provided some more thorough exams, and our options were limited. Her back leg was broken beyond repair. She ended up having her back leg amputated. She also had several injuries in her ribs and other internal organs. She had a serious wound on her stomach. After a day or two at the vet, we brought her home, hoping she could recover.

The next few days were rough. She could not walk. She would not eat or drink anything. I had to carry her outside to see if she would even try to go to the bathroom. She would not. I slept on the floor with her and had to change the bandage on her stomach every four hours or so.

Duder did not know how to react to any of this either. Daisy would not let Duder near her; she would growl at him. You could see the sadness in his eyes.

After a week, it was clear that she was not going to recover. We had to make a decision. I took her to the vet, and we put her down. I then took her out to the trails where we spent our time together. I found a spot and buried her so she would always be in her happy place.

Got me thinking...

This was a very hard experience for the Blonde and me—much harder than I would have imagined. This silly little dog had become a big part of our lives, and now she was gone. We had to grieve. We had to accept. We had to try and move on. This is true of any kind of loss in our lives. What we learned is that you cannot let things like this destroy you. You must find a way to accept and move on

Duder didn't understand what happened to Dasiy. For the next few months, he would spend time wandering around, looking for her. He wanted his friend back. I wish I could have explained this to him. He had to accept her loss in his own way.

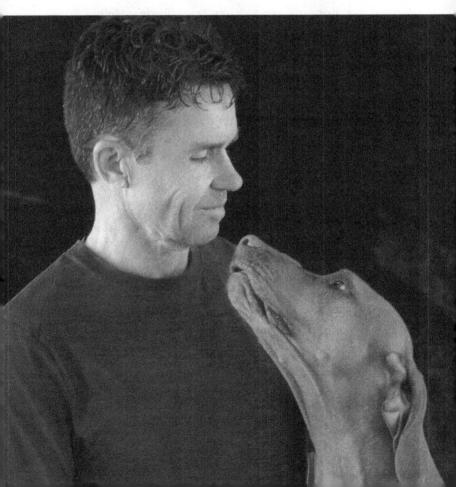

MY THREE FAVORITE COLORS

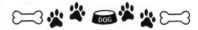

I can honestly say that my three favorite colors are blue, green, and brown. These are the colors Duder and I see on the trail. The blue sky, the green trees and grass, and the beautiful brown dirt.

This became our happy place. Both of us love the trails. Being outside in the fresh air, absorbing the sounds and smells of nature, and soaking in the beauty of it all. It is good for the soul.

Got me thinking...

Do we have a happy place in our minds? Is there somewhere we can close our eyes and go to that will provide some peace?

I have had times in my life where that happy place was hard to find. Maybe we have all been there. Life takes over, then stress, anxiety, and anguish can overtake us.

I have found that being able to find and go to our own internal happy place is critical for a healthy life. Techniques can be used to do this: meditation, yoga, gratitude journals, affirmations etc. We all need to find what works for us.

For me, heading out to the trail and focusing on the blue, green, and brown was my form of meditation. On the trails, I didn't worry about anything else; I could just observe the colors and truly appreciate the moment. That was, and continues to be, my happy place.

DUDER HAS NO REGRETS

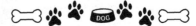

Duder will sometimes do something that he either knows he shouldn't do, or that he soon wishes he didn't do. He will get into trouble by me or be stuck somewhere that he does not want to be.

What I have noticed is that once the event is over, he is able to learn from the moment, but he is back to his normal tail-wagging self very quickly. He does not dwell.

Got me thinking...

When I hit fifty years old and Duder and I would head out for our daily walk, I would spend a great deal of time thinking about the past. I thought about my life as a spouse, a father, a son, and a grandfather. When I thought about the past, regrets would naturally come to mind: I wish I had done this, I wish I hadn't done that. Why wasn't I a better father? What was I thinking when I did that?

Our minds are always cranking with ideas and

thoughts, and when these thoughts are negative, they can be very debilitating. They came at me hard, especially at this milestone of fifty years old.

I had to find a way to not let these thoughts control me and dictate my future. My mindset had to change.

To change my mindset, I had to start with my self-talk. When I would go on walks with Duder, I would constantly talk to myself. I purposefully forced my self-talk to change. "Do not focus on the past." "What are you going to do today?" "What will your tomorrow look like?"

Over time, I concluded that I cannot change the past. I had to come to terms with that idea, accept it, and implement it. This meant that I could no longer let the past control me. My "past self" talking in my head had to shut up. He was annoying.

My "future self" had to control my internal dialogue. I can only control what I think, say, and do from this second on. Mindset changed to consciously thinking of my future.

My biggest regrets had to do with the Blonde and my kids. Many of the regrets were set pretty deep. I cannot change the past. It doesn't matter how sorry or bad I felt at the time. It doesn't even matter how many times I apologized or if I continue to apologize to this day. What matters is what I do now—my actions. I now do different things. I want the Blonde and my kids to see me doing different things. I want them to see me moving forward in life with a new view and perspective, and a refreshed appreciation for having them in my life.

My regrets still exist, they always will. I can't change the past, though, and reminding myself of that is the key to moving forward.

DUDER AND HIS BLADDER

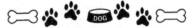

When we are in the house and we do not have access to a doggy door, Duder will go and stand by the door to let us know he needs to go out and take care of business. At one point, we even put a small bell by the door. Sometimes if we ignore him and don't open the door the instant he demands it, he will either give up and go sit down somewhere, or he will start barking at us. When he really needs to go, he will start to wiggle around, doing the potty dance (the Blonde is good at this dance as well). He is looking at us and begging us with his eyes and body to OPEN THE DOOR!!

Got me thinking...

I was fifty years old when this all started. I am fifty-five now. During this phase, I needed to create the same sense of urgency that Duder had when he needed that door opened. I am old. I am running out of time. I will not live forever.

One thing I did was create a life grid. It was a piece

of paper with 100 squares, each one representing a year of life. Each square had twelve small boxes representing each month in the year. I took a blue pen and colored in the first years and months of my life up until I got married. I then marked every month after that with green. I now mark every month as it passes with the green.

This gave me a visual representation of my life. The boxes are running out. Am I going to live to be 100? If not, then the remaining boxes will be even fewer.

Just looking at this grid and seeing my time running out gave me the sense of urgency that I needed. If I'm going to accomplish everything that I want to, then I better get started!

FINDING RENEWAL WITH CHANGE

A period of time after losing Daisy, we decided to bring another member into our family. Welcome Roxie. She is a Weimaraner puppy. She is different than Daisy. She is a bit more obnoxious. She is trying to be the alpha dog in the house, and Duder does not like that. She has now grown to be bigger than Duder and pretty much controls the situation. The two of them are still working out how they will live together.

She is a change in all of our lives.

Got me thinking...

Sometimes a way to deal with loss and change is to introduce more change to the situation. It doesn't erase our loss, but it helps us move from stagnation; it urges us forward.

We loved Daisy, and we will never forget her. At the same time, Roxie now has a place in our hearts, and we will love her for who she is.

PUPPY PHASE, ALL OVER AGAIN.

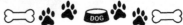

Here we go again—it's puppy phase all over. Roxie is a stubborn little pup, chewing and peeing everywhere. Sheesh. The training is tough, the patience required is hard to find, and the overall experience of a puppy can be hard.

Not sure what is harder: the training of the puppy or training the Blonde to train the new puppy.

Got me thinking...

New things are hard, and changes in life can be stressful. It took some time, but I have learned to embrace it—in fact, I learned to seek it out. A change is what I was after when I hit fifty. I decided that I needed to do things differently, and as a result, I've been able to transform myself. I now choose to dive in head first, be diligent, and love the change.

For example, I started a new job a while ago. I knew it would be difficult on me and the Blonde to adapt to this new routine and to learn these new things. I made a very conscious choice to do my best in the new role. I set some very specific personal goals that I wanted to achieve; this helped me get into the mindset that was needed. I also renewed my mindset daily, consistently shifting my focus back to my goals. Because of this, when things got tough, I was able to push through and come out of the tough and stressful days with good results.

The Blonde and I set some goals and basic guidelines to put in place for Roxie's training. We have not met them all (mostly because Roxie is a stubborn Weimaraner. We sometime refer to her as BB—barky bitch).

The lesson is to embrace any change, get your mindset in proper place, set your aspirations of how to move forward, and stick to them always.

DUDER SLEEPS A LOT

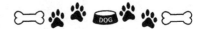

"You will perform better, make better decisions, and have a better body when you get the sleep you require."
—Shawn Stevenson, The Model Health Show

During a normal day, Duder is typically a very active dog. He loves to run and he needs his exercise. He is always wondering what the Blonde and I are doing, and whatever is it, he wants to do it with us. But, if there is nothing going on, he will always lay down and sleep. He sleeps a lot.

Got me thinking...

In my transformation, it became clear to me early on how important sleep was. It affected most things in my life: my weight, my running, my mental state, my focus, my discipline—you name it, good or bad sleep will impact it.

There is an abundance of studies and research on sleep and its importance. I started to do some research on my own sleep patterns, and I realized that I did not have good sleep habits. I started to incorporate some changes in my sleep. Here are some simple things I changed:

- I stopped taking my phone or tablet to bed with me. Instead, I left them in the other room.
- I made my room as dark as possible. I put tape over the little light coming from the smoke detector, and I turned off the clock in the room. The room I sleep in is very dark and quiet.
- I created consistency. I go to bed at 8:30 p.m. every day—yes, every day—and I read a book for twenty to thirty minutes before I go to sleep.
- I wake up at 5:00 a.m. No snoozing. I simply get out of bed and drink a glass of water.
- My target is eight hours of sleep per night, and sticking to my sleep schedule ensures that.
- It was important for me to have these very specific habits. Over time, my mind and body adapted to this. Every night at 8:30, I start to shut down; my body tells me to go to bed. I don't have to set an alarm anymore; I am naturally able to wake up around 5:00 a.m.
- In the morning, I do simple resistance training: HIIT or basic yoga. Then I do my daily run.

As I incorporated these sleep habits, I noticed changes in how my body responded. I had more energy. I did not feel tired in the morning. My mind was more alert and less foggy. My most productive hours in a day have been from 5:00 to 8:00 a.m. This is also when I would write this

DUDER'S CHALLENGE

What are your current sleep patterns? Record them, as well as other habits you have that impact your sleep. What are some improvements and changes you can make? Try to set a schedule for every night and day of when you go to sleep and wake up. Make it a priority so you can be the most efficient you possible.

WHERE SHOULD DUDER SLEEP?

There are many opinions about where dogs should sleep. Put them in a kennel, have them sleep on their own bed, let them sleep on my bed, or maybe even in the bathtub?

Duder sleeps in my bed with me. Yes, he sleeps with me.

Got me thinking...

The Blonde and I have been married for thirty-seven years. As I began doing things differently, the two of us acknowledged that we have different sleep patterns and habits. I started going to bed early and waking up early. The Blonde does not.

For the sanity of both of us, we made a choice to sleep in separate rooms. She has her space and I have mine. She has her own routines and I have mine. This might sound weird, but having been married for so long, it actually works pretty well for us. When my wife gets a good night's sleep, it is good for her, and a happy wife equals a happy life. So, she needed me out of her room and routine as much I needed her out of mine.

I would not recommend this for all couples. When you have been married, let's say, for at least thirty-five years, then you can consider this. Until then, it is important for couples to sleep together; that time is when you truly grow up together and live your life together.

DUDER SLEEPS AROUND

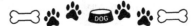

There are occasions where we need to find a boarder to take care of the dogs while the Blonde and I are out vacationing or visiting family.

We have tried the big dog boarding places; we have also found some local families that board dogs in their homes. On one occasion, we needed to board the dogs for two nights with a local family. When we picked the dogs up after their stay, they told us that Roxie slept in her kennel, but Duder slept with them—with the new people, in their bed, with them.

Say what? Duder was sleeping around on me!!

Got me thinking...

When the Blonde and I first started sleeping in separate rooms, and Duder started sleeping in my bed, it caused a little strife. She was jealous of him. I would rather sleep with him than her. This is weird for me to even type this out.

When we heard where Duder was sleeping at the

boarder's place, I had a better understanding of what the Blonde was feeling.

The Blonde no longer feels this way. She enjoys not having my stinky, snoring, constantly hot, and restless body in her bed.

ENVIRONMENT

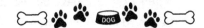

There are times when Duder will be tired or bored and I am not giving him any attention, so, he will look for a place to lay down, maybe take a nap. Sometimes, he will climb onto his doggy bed, but he will adjust it. He will stand on it and walk around in circles. He will also fluff it up in certain areas by pawing at it. He will lay down, for a second, but it is not quite right, so he will stand up and start the routine over again. He will do this until everything is just right, and only then can he lay down.

Got me thinking...

What is my environment like? Do I need to make adjustments to make it just right? Should I spin around in my living room?

One of the first things I did in my transformation journey was cancel my satellite TV subscription. One day, I walked into the living room and realized that the focus of the room was the TV. Each of us must decide for ourselves if that is what we want. I made a choice that the TV and its focus were not good for me or the Blonde.

When I did not have access to TV anymore, my view of the world changed. I was not worried about when the game was on. I did not care about certain shows anymore. I was not watching the mainstream news anymore. I was not taking in all the commercials anymore. The Blonde was no longer taking these things in as often either, so we began doing other things both together and separately. Going for walks. Reading. Learning. And yes, talking to each other.

DUDER'S CHALLENGE

There are so many other things that might need some changing in your environment. Take a look at where you live, your work environment, your car, places you go to and hang out at, and the people you surround yourself with. Are these all good for you?

Be like Duder: Spin around in your environment and look at everything around you. Evaluate. Adjust as needed.

FASCINATION WITH POOP

Sometimes while out on the trails, Duder and I come across some poop of another animal. And, of course, Duder has to stop to check it out, smell it, and maybe even eat some of it.

I don't understand the dog's fascination with poop. For most of us, poop is gross and we don't want anything to do with it.

Got me thinking...

On occasion, when we are out on the trails, I'll need to stop and use one of the trail bathrooms. These are typically no-flush outhouses—which is just a big hole to collect everyone's waste. Anyone that has ever used one of these knows that they are not a pleasant experience. Have you ever had the urge or the need to look inside the toilet? Kind of like Duder checking out the horse poop? Have you ever done it? I have. And no, I don't do it anymore. That is an image that I do not want to keep with me.

But, why in the world would I look inside that thing? Do I just want to see what everyone's poop looks like? Is it natural human curiosity? How does having that information—or in this case, that image—help me in any way?

The lesson is about our inputs. What inputs are you welcoming into your mind and existence? Inputs come in many forms, such as TV shows and movies. It's the question of content you seek out. What are you looking at on the internet? What kind of video games do you play? Do you read books or listen to podcasts? What kind of music do you listen to? What type of people do you interact with, and what are common things that they say?

I changed my inputs. I began reading books and listening to informative podcasts. I stopped watching TV and greatly reduced my time on social media.

I learned that what you put into your mind greatly impacts what comes out of it. It impacts your internal thoughts and your external interactions with the world.

DUDER'S CHALLENGE

So, with every input, ask yourself this question: Is it Poop? Are you inputting the bottom of that porta potty? It might be time to truly evaluate what you are putting into your mind. All inputs will have an impact. Decide which ones help you and hurt you.

RUNNING IN THE DARK

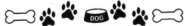

During the fall and winter months, the sun takes its time coming up in the mornings. Duder and I are early morning runners. Many of our runs are done in the darkness, so I need to wear a headlamp. Duder must have much better eyes than me, because he doesn't need a headlamp and has no problem navigating the trails in the darkness.

Sometimes, the runs in the dark are my favorite. The trails are empty and it is very quiet and peaceful in the early mornings.

Side Note: Last year, I participated in a half-marathon race called "Zion at Night." I was very happy that my youngest daughter completed the race with me. This was a trail race completed during the night, under the stars. We had a great time.

During these dark runs, I could only see as far as my headlamp would shine. Beyond that, it was complete darkness. I could not see behind me and had very limited visibility to my sides. Duder would take off down the trail, well beyond my headlamp. Then at some point, I would see two very faint red dots in the darkness. That was Duder stopping to make sure I was still coming. (At least, I would hope it was Duder, but who knows what other animals were out there.)

Got me thinking...

The limited distance that I could see did not stop me from running ahead. I had to have some faith that the trail would continue and that I would not fall off the mountain. I was truly in a small little bubble of existence; I did not know what else was around me.

I realized that a big chunk of my life was like I was living in that bubble, not able to see what was beyond the headlamp. I was only interested in and processing the inputs from that small little world.

My transformation started. I started learning. I started reading. I brought more input into my world. I started trying new things. I put myself out into the world. Each of these small steps made the light on my life's headlamp shine a little bit brighter and reach a little farther. I had a much clearer view of what was ahead, what was around me, and what was possible.

I was no longer living in the dark; I was living in the light that I created.

COUNTER SURFING

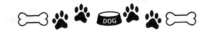

"If you don't risk anything, you risk even more." —Erika Jong

A common behavior that a lot of dog owners must deal with is counter surfing. Duder will come into the kitchen and always wonder what's on the counter. He can usually smell something. When we are with him, he behaves and doesn't jump up on the counter. He will sit there and look at us, urging us to give him some food. So, he knows he is not supposed to jump up on the counter. He knows he will get into trouble.

Now, what about the times when we are not in the kitchen with him? There are times when a loaf of bread somehow goes missing. That cube of butter is gone— butter is one of his absolute favorite foods to steal. He has even taken big bites out of a chocolate cake.

I have been in the other room and observed Duder in the kitchen. I have watched him look around to see if we are close. He will then take some sniffs to try and evaluate what might be up on the counter. It is almost like he is pondering the consequences of grabbing the item, weighing the pros and cons. Will it be worth it? Is it worth the risk?

Got me thinking...

Over my life, I can remember things that were on the counter that were out of my immediate reach. These might've been physical things, or goals I wanted to achieve—maybe items on my bucket list. In the past, I was not able to push myself past this idea of "risk" to jump up and get those things I wanted. Risk, for me, was getting out of my comfort zone and putting myself out into the world. I avoided doing this because I'd be worried about what people would think of me. These concerns were very real to me. I truly did spend time evaluating whether the reward was worth the risk.

But at some point, I decided that I wanted what was on the counter. I was willing to do whatever it took to jump up and grab it, regardless of the consequences. I felt like Duder; that cube of butter was worth the risk to him, and putting myself out there was worth it to me.

And you know what? I don't even get all that mad at Duder for counter surfing anymore. He inspires me.

CHASING THAT RABBIT

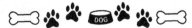

Duder loves to chase rabbits; out on our hikes, he was always looking for them. When he would see one, he'd take off, chasing that rabbit wherever it went. To this day, he has never caught one.

One time, we were hiking next to a steep mountain and we were down in the valley portion. A rabbit was sniffed out and discovered early on, so Duder began his quest after it. The rabbit ran straight up the side of the mountain, and Duder followed suit. It was hard for him to run straight up, but he gave it his best. Eventually, he had to stop. The rabbit was long gone, and Duder was too tired to go on.

Got me thinking...

During my transformation, there were so many things I was doing differently, and my mindset was changing as a result. At one point, I wrote down a list of personal affirmations on my whiteboard. Some of them were things like, "I am a runner," "I am writer," and "I am a great husband."

One that I really liked and embraced was: "I am a badass." It is up to interpretation what a badass is, but how I envisioned it was a person who did badass things, like running marathons and ultramarathons. This is part of why I like to do those hard things—because I am a badass!!

This would translate into my training runs. Sometimes while I was out on a trail run, there'd be a steep hill that I had to climb. I would think of Duder; if he can do it, then so can I. I am a badass, I have to run up this steep hill!!

However, I found that this way of thinking wasn't sustainable, and it soon needed to change. As I began doing longer runs and much more climbing up mountains, I had to develop some smarter behaviors. I did some research, talked with some running friends, and realized that I needed to make my long runs as efficient as possible. On the very steep climbs, it is more efficient to power hike instead of run. This gets you to the top in almost the same amount of time, but you won't be as tired when you get there.

In essence, I had to become a smart badass. I needed to run smarter. This also applied to other things, such as work, relationships, projects, and even writing. I found ways to be more effective and efficient. If there are two different ways to get to the same place in the same amount of time, why would you choose the path that'd make you twice as tired?

I am now a smart badass...Does that make me a smartass?

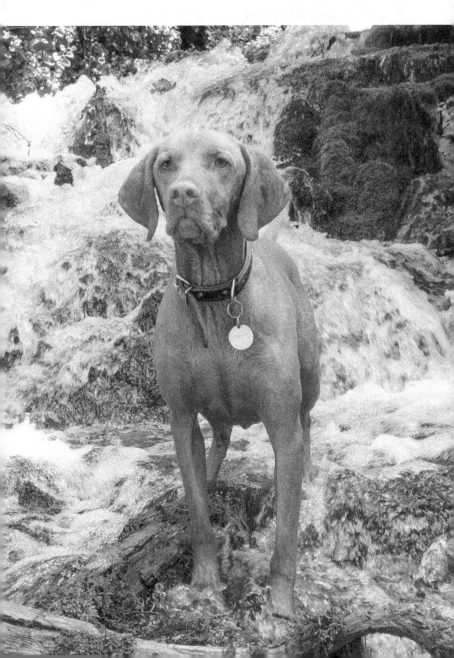

DUDER AND HIS BONE

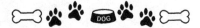

Sometimes we would give Duder a raw bone from the butcher, and we'd also give Roxie one. They both became very protective of their bones. If Roxie showed any sign that she wanted Duder's bone, he would react and growl at her. Tensions were always high when the bones were in play.

Many times, Duder would go out and bury his bone outside. Yes, this is a real thing. When he had one buried out there, he always wanted to go outside to check on it. Even Roxie would go out to find Duder's bone and check on it. There were times when it felt like all they could think about was that stupid bone.

Got me thinking...

When you are eighteen and married, you have to learn about money very quickly. Whether you like it or not, money is required in our world. You learn good and bad ways to manage your money and incomes. Sometimes money felt like that stupid bone—obsessing over it, being constantly worried about it, and always checking on it.

Through our thirty-seven years of marriage, the Blond and I have had a mixed relationship with money. Sometimes the topic has caused a great deal of strife between us.

Back in 1998, I started a new job working for a start-up company. They offered me a salary and some stock options. The stock options were then converted to full stock in vesting exercises over four years. Soon after I started working there, the company climbed aboard the dot-com boom and decided to make themselves a publicly traded company. My stock options went from a value of about fifty cents a share to over twenty bucks a share in a single day. They were still options and not yet vested, so I could not realize any cash value. Over a period of about six months, the public stock price kept going up. It spiked in price during a short period, and I was a millionaire—at least, my unvested stock options were valued at over a million. The Blonde and I had it made. Woohoo!!

But then...

The dot-com crash happened. Stock prices tumbled. My company exploded, and not in a good way. Half the employees were laid off, including me. My options were no good. The brokerage sent me a check with the final value of my options. I have this check hanging on my wall in my office. It is a check for $0.01. Yes, they sent me a one cent check.

I went to work for a different company soon after and

they were not doing any better. I was shortly laid off from that one as well.

Our finances were not in good shape at this point. We were stuck in a situation where we could not find a way out. We ended up filing for bankruptcy.

I have not told many people about the bankruptcy. It is a painful time that I do not like to think about.

The lesson is that money is important. Methods and plans to manage your money effectively are even more important. You never know what is going to happen. Teach your kids.

Maybe burying your money in the backyard is not a good idea.

DUDER IS NOT SHY

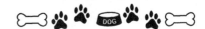

Duder will say hello to anyone that will give him even the slightest bit of attention. He is not shy whatsoever. He is too much for some people, but this is his normal behavior. We have spent some time training him to be a little calmer, not to jump on people, not to lick everyone's faces. We have not been very good at this, but we are working on it.

Got me thinking...

For most of my life, I would say that my normal behavior was more on the shy and introverted side of things. As my transformation began and small changes in my mindset began to settle in, this has changed.

Also, I realized that if I was going to write this book, I would need to display my truest self, and everyone who reads this book would then know me. So, I needed to put myself out there. I embraced the idea of telling my story and letting others see it.

Part of my goal for writing this book is to inspire others that may need some changes in their lives. How do I reach those people that are sitting on their couch right now, watching TV with no interest in reading a book. This is a question I am still pondering. That person is who I used to be. I was not reading self-help books. I was not listening to podcasts. I was not listening to inspirational speakers. How did someone reach me?

Duder took me out of my comfort zone. He brought me out into the world. I am meeting new people, I am engaged in new activities, and I am trying to play a bigger role in my community.

I am fifty-five years old. It is never too late to make a change.

BEING PRESENT

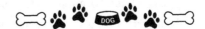

The Blonde and I love to take the pups out and explore new places. Living in Utah, we have explored some of the coolest places on our great blue planet. The Blonde really loves the waterfalls. We'd search for them and schedule adventures to go and see them. She had to get the cool pictures with the dogs for the Instagram page.

When we plan these adventures, they always include a hike. The four of us heading out on the trails became part of who we all are. We all love it. What I realized is that the longer the hike was, the more "in tune" with the hike we became. All the other things going on in the world and in our lives just faded away, and we would become present with the land, the trail, the water, and each other.

Got me thinking...

When you are not on a hike and you are going about your daily routines and business, it is hard, very hard, to be present. There are so many distractions—the biggest one for most of us is probably our stupid phones. Our minds have grown so restless that we cannot focus on anything anymore.

I have tried to make very specific adjustments in my behavior to make myself more present in my life. I am aware that there are times that I am not present. I can be with someone and even be having a conversation with them, but I am not there; my mind is somewhere else. Once you are aware that you might be behaving like this, you can start to incorporate techniques to change this.

To repair my relationship with the Blonde, I needed to make a critical behavior change and actually become present while with her.

Here are some things we both try and practice:

- We eat dinner together, and no phones are allowed at the table—and I don't mean that we set our phones face-down on the table. Phones are not allowed anywhere in sight.
- We limit our TV time. This took a little getting used to, but we very quickly learned that you do not have to watch TV every day. You can go days without it.
- We share the podcasts and books that we are listening to or reading, and we discuss what we've learned and what we find interesting within them.
- I ask her about her day and actually listen—I don't cut her off with a response; I just listen.

DUDER'S CHALLENGE

Take some time and ask yourself if you are as present as you could be in your relationships. Does something need to change?

Make a list of your priorities. Then make a second list of what your priorities actually are based on your current actions. Does your actions' priority list look like this?

- Phone
- Social Media
- TV Shows
- Sports
- Alcohol
- Partner

If so, then you may need some changes. How can you move your partner to the top of your priority list?

CARRYING DUDER'S POOP

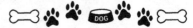

On the days when I would take Duder and Roxie out on a morning road run, Duder would always have to stop to mark his territory by peeing on all the trees and bushes. But Roxie would only occasionally pee on our runs. Very strange.

I would also have to put the doggy poop bags in my pocket, and Duder would always have to stop to take his dump. We would wait, I would pull out the poop bag, then I'd pick up his poop. I would then need to carry this poop bag until we found a garbage can. So, here I am, trying to run, carrying around this warm and smelly bag of dog poop.

Got me thinking...

The Blonde maintains an Instagram page for the pups. The process of posting on these social media platforms can be frustrating. She has a different kind of phone than I do, and her phone would give her problems with the process. In these cases, she would use my phone to make a post. The other day, she was using my phone to post a reel. My phone did not have access to the same emojis as hers. This made her angry, because she needed those emojis on the post!! She lashed out at me. It was my fault that my phone did not have what she needed! She wanted to get it posted by a certain time! She didn't have her hashtags ready! She was running out of time!!!

In that moment, as she was projecting this all onto me, I felt like I was carrying around a bag of her poop. Why did I have to carry her poop?

As with Duder, the sooner I can find that garbage can and get rid of that bag, the better. The same thing applied with the Blonde: I can carry that poop for a while, but the sooner I get rid of it, the better. I can't keep it with me, can't fester over it, and can't react to it. I need to let it go and dump it in the nearest garbage can.

LEAF PATROL

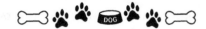

Duder loves the wind. If the wind is blowing, there are usually leaves and other things blowing around. Duder will hear the wind come up and will have to go outside—I call it going on leaf patrol. He's the one in charge of chasing every one of those pesky little things and making sure they are not causing anyone any problems. He'll lay down outside and be on full alert until the wind stops or it starts raining.

Got me thinking...

I used to be a big fan of sports. I followed a lot of different sports and loved to follow the news, the trades, all the things happening with a league. My go-to sport was basketball, specifically the NBA, and being from Utah, I had my team that I followed. I used to be a little crazy about it. At one point, I was keeping my own spreadsheet with information about them. I tracked scores, news, and stats on a daily basis. I listened to sports on the radio and watched sports on TV. I loved to sit down and watch the game. I was in full-blown leaf patrol.

Then, I started my transformation. I turned the TV off, which meant no more watching sports. That was rough. I started to bring different and new inputs into my world. The importance of sports faded away with time. Other things started to be more important, such as my family and, in particular, the Blonde. I still check the scores occasionally and keep track of my team, but I am no longer obsessed with it like I used to be. I realized that the time I was spending focusing on it was not bringing me any value.

The point is that there are things we put too much of our time and energy into that do not bring value to our lives.

DUDER'S CHALLENGE

Your time is more valuable than anything else, so take a moment to assess where you're currently spending your time and energy. When you have done that, go through each item on the list and truly ask yourself if it is helping you. Is anything causing strife within your job? Your relationships? Your physical wellbeing?

If they are not moving you forward, then find the tools and techniques to eliminate them from your life.

DUDER, STOP DOING THAT!!

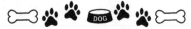

Over the years that Duder has been with us, he has had a few injuries. Some of these include a scrape or a gouge in his paw. At one point, we discovered that he was missing a small chunk of his ear. We have no idea how that happened, but we suspect Roxie had something to do with it.

Duder must have stepped on a rock or branch while out on the trail one time, because he came home with a cut on one of his paws. As is the norm for dogs with something like this, he was obsessed with that cut. He kept licking it, over and over again. We would try to get him to stop, but he would always go back to it.

Got me thinking...

When I think about my running journey, I have had people comment all kinds of things to me. Some of them positive, some of them not. Things like, "Are you crazy?" "Why would do you do that?" "You shouldn't do that; you'll hurt your knees," and "You are going to damage your heart." Each of these comments came from non-runners.

This is not just about running. Anything you do, there will always be someone making negative comments about it. It might be directly from a person you know, a post on social media, or even a commercial on the TV.

If you let it, these ideas and thoughts can really affect you. They can shut you down and make you want to go back into your comfort zone, the place where you are doing nothing to make people react this way towards you. I used to be there, and I admit, it's easier to stay inside that safe bubble you form around yourself.

However, once you start and engage in something that exposes yourself to those around you, you better have a plan to deal and cope with the negative side of things. You need to think through what will come and prepare yourself on how you will respond. If you have envisioned the scenario in your mind and have visualized your response, then it won't knock you down.

SUCCESS

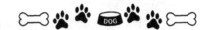

When we first brought Duder home as a puppy, we began the process of training him. He had to learn where to pee and poop and where to sleep, and he slowly learned the rules of the house. During this process, he learned very quickly that if he walked to the back door, he was telling us that he needed to go out. The first time this happened was a fantastic success—no more pee in the house!

Got me thinking...

I really had to reevaluate my understanding and interpretation of success.

The rich folks out there (or the ones who seem to have a lot of money) always seem to get that label of "successful." Did I have to have a lot of money to be successful? Was that the only way? Surely there was another way, I rationalized, and then began my work towards becoming a "successful" person.

This started with my simple commitment to waking up early. Inspired by Jocko Willink, I decided that 5:00 a.m. was a good time to start my day. So, this habit began back then and continues to this day. I wake up at 5:00, go look myself in the mirror, then congratulate myself on my success. This allowed me to start each and every day with a success that would lead to the next item that I considered successful. I would say that 99.9% of my successes happen silently; they are my own successes and no one else needs to know about them.

Every time I sat down to write, it was a success. Every time the Blonde and I spend some quality time together, success. Every run, every bed I make, every day with no sugar, every time I work out—all of those things fill my days with success.

DUDER'S CHALLENGE

What does success mean to you? There might be different definitions based on where you're applying it, but focus on the small first. What does success look like within your relationships, your personal endeavors, and in your daily life?

Find your little accomplishments in every day, and make sure you give yourself credit for them.

HOW FAST IS DUDER?

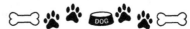

Duder is a Vizsla, and Daisy was a Vizsla as well. This breed is listed as one of the fastest dogs among all breeds and can reach speeds up to 40 mph. A Weimaraner, which is Roxie's breed, is also among one of the fastest breeds; although they're not quite as fast as Vizslas, they can reach speeds up to 35 mph. We have some fast dogs in our house.

Watching them run is always cool. They love to run. When Daisy started running, we noticed that she was much faster than Duder. When Roxie came along, she was faster than Duder as well. Duder could still move pretty well, but I guess he is on the slow side of his breed. That did not stop him from running though.

Got me thinking...

I remember a day early on in my transformation when Duder and I were out hiking on a trail, and for some strange reason, I just started running. I ran for about 100 yards before I was out of breath. I remember thinking,

"Hmm, maybe I can do this." This is how my running journey got started.

I then remember running my first two miles without stopping. It really was a momentous occasion. At some point, something clicked, and I decided I wanted to do more. I signed up for a half marathon. I then figured out a training plan and went to work in executing it. When I finished the first half marathon, it was a big deal for me.

Whenever people heard that I ran a race, the question most of them asked was: "What was your time?" In some ways, this got annoying. I didn't care about my time—the fact that I was doing it at all was what mattered to me. But then I fell into the speed trap for future races. During other half marathons, I started getting worried about my times, how I placed in my age group, and how I placed overall.

What I learned is that I am like Duder. I am on the slow side of my breed. I am not a fast runner and will most likely never be on the podium. After running more races, I concluded that I am not doing it for the time; I am doing it because I can, and I am damn proud of myself for running these events and distances at my age. I will still check the results to see my times, but I am no longer trying to set a personal best. I love the atmosphere of organized races. I love meeting people like me who are also there to torture themselves. I am running the races to keep me motivated and for the experience.

I am happy to be in the race.

Learning that I wasn't the fastest in races was really helpful to me because it applied to other things I was working on. I was doing many things that were new to me, and I decided that, like my running, I don't need to be the best at those things. I just want to be in the race; I just wanted to experience new things and push myself. I have concluded that it is better to be in the race than on the sidelines wishing you were out there.

CHALLENGES

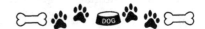

"Today might be the best chance you have to take action. The longer you wait, the more deeply embedded you get in your current lifestyle. Your habits solidify. Your beliefs harden. You get comfortable. It will never be easy, but it may also never be easier than it is right now."
—James Clear

Duder and I have taken some long hikes and runs together. We have both reached points of extreme exhaustion. I have seen Duder find a stream and just lay down in it. He will rest for a while, but he will always get up and keep going.

Got me thinking...

As I started running more races, I started to get a pretty cool collection of medals. One year for Christmas, my middle daughter made me a wooden holder where I could hang my medals. On the board, she wrote this saying: "If it doesn't challenge you, it doesn't change you." As I was going through my transformation, everything was changing—I was changing myself. I embraced this idea that if I wanted change, then I needed to challenge myself.

Challenge comes in many forms. When you do anything different than you normally would, this can be challenging.

Let's start with running. When I was fifty, I was overweight and had a hard time even walking for half a mile. So, that first walk with Duder was out of my normal routine and was a challenge for me. I remember hiking on the trail one day while I was still losing weight, and I did my first 100 yard run—that was all I could do. That 100 yards was a challenge. I then remember the first time I ran two miles without stopping. I was damn proud of myself. I even bragged to my kids and wife! It was the hardest two miles I have ever run. I think that was as challenging as my first half marathon. It had a huge impact on me. It started to plant some ideas in my head of what was possible. If I could do that, then what else could I do?

I decided then to continue to challenge myself. I signed up for a half marathon and began the next leg of my running journey. As I trained, I started to add more miles and do longer runs. Each progressively longer run continued to challenge me, my mind, my legs, and my lungs. At one point, I remember having the thought that I was happy with running half marathons, but after running enough of them, I decided that the half wasn't as big of a challenge as it used to be. I needed to up my game, so I signed up for a marathon. This then expanded to a couple of ultramarathons, with more of them planned afterwards. I found that the runs were very symbolic for me. I used the idea of challenging myself in my runs as a mechanism to challenge myself with other aspects of my life.

A big part of transformation is in your mind. Being able to change the way you think is challenging. When I started to think about my relationship with the Blonde, I had to make some serious adjustments on my side and to my part. I had to own up to what I did and the role I played. This was new thinking for me. I was used to just coasting along and blaming her for everything. I had to practice being aware of what I was doing, but before I was able to practice, I needed to first make the conscious decision to change. It was like my running: I had to get that first 100 yard run in first, then the rest would become easier. It takes time, commitment, and practice.

This idea of change and challenge is critical for any transformation you want to make. If you want something different, then you have to do something different.

DUDER'S CHALLENGE

Mind. Meal. Move. Find something different in each of these areas to start to challenge yourself. Some ideas might be:

- Mind: Turn off the TV one night a week.
- Meal: Skip that beer or glass of wine you want to have.
- Move: Park in the farthest parking spot away from the store so you must walk.

These are simple things, but they might be different than normal routines, so they might be slightly challenging. Starting small is okay, because every small step can lead to other, bigger changes.

Change will not come without challenge.

DUDER AND I HAVE THE SAME BIRTHDAY 🐾 🦴

When we first decided we wanted a puppy, we looked around at different litters. We found a litter that was born on the same day as me. I saw a picture of Duder from the litter and I knew that we were meant to be together.

On November 21, 2021, Duder turned five, and I turned fifty-four. In "dog years," Duder was about thirty-five. He was, and still is, in his prime. Still very active. Still running. Still very healthy. But that will change, and I know that Duder's life will be shorter than mine.

Dogs just do not live as long as their humans—that's just the way it is. It's a sad thought, but I will enjoy his company for as long as I have him.

Got me thinking...

When should I retire? What is my life span? How long do I have left?

In my overall life, I am currently in the best physical shape I've ever been in. After losing weight, building endurance, and making efforts to become a more thoughtful and educated person, I am proud of who I've become. But birthdays always have a way of triggering thoughts and reflection.

The world tries to tell you that you have a finite time of being productive in the world. That you need to plan your finances so you can retire by fifty-five, and that afterwards, you will only relax and do nothing—maybe just the occasional golf game or visit with the grandkids.

At some point in life, you reach a certain age and have some natural thoughts like, "I'm too old to start anything new," and "I should have done it earlier; there's no use starting now."

Well, SCREW those ideas. I no longer believe in the idea of retirement. It's a stupid concept. I have no intention of ever retiring.

I started my transformation at fifty years old. It is never too late. NEVER.

On that Sunday morning, November 21, 2021, I turned fifty-four years old. It was 5:00 a.m. It was 25°F outside. I woke up and thought about going back to bed. It was my birthday, so I deserved it. But I looked back on everything I had learned over the previous three years, and all the knowledge and experiences kicked in. I got up, looked at myself in the mirror, and imagined I was looking at "Old Age." I said out loud, "SCREW YOU, OLD AGE! I am just getting started. You are not going to stop me!" I put my running gear on and went out for a fifteen-mile run, all the while laughing at Old Age.

It is never too late. If something needs to change in your life, change it. Do it today.

WHY DOES DUDER RUN?

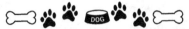

"Tomorrow becomes never. No matter how small the task, take the
first step now!" –Tim Ferriss

From the time when we brought Duder home to us
as a puppy, he always wanted to run wherever he went.
There was very little casual walking; it was always run,
run, run. Running is just a natural part of a dog's life.

Got me thinking...

As I was going through my transformation journey,
I moved into a learning and writing mode. I was always
looking for ideas and nuggets of information. Obviously,
I found knowledge in analogies.

When I was out on my morning runs, my mind would
always be looking for these ideas, and I would usually
come up with running analogies. This is a list of some of
the running analogies and lessons learned that came to
me. These applied specifically to my running, but these
ideas can be applied to any aspect of life.

Think about a project you are working on, or a
relationship you want to improve, do these ideas apply?

- Running towards something. I would put a vision of something out there, a view of my future self or something I wanted, and that is what I was running towards.

- Running away from something. I was always running away from my past self. Sometimes I would think about my age: mid-fifties. I wanted to run away from my age.

- How far to run? I used to have a detailed training plan that said I needed to run five miles on this day and three miles on that day. So, on that five-mile run, I would run five miles. There were times that I would feel good and could run farther, but because I set my target at five, that was all I would do. I found this to be limiting. I started to change the wording when setting my goals. For example, instead of "Run five miles," it is now, "Run *at least* five miles." Then, if I am feeling good and my legs are moving well, I would run for longer. I stopped limiting myself.

- Running uphill. Running up a hill is hard, which is why I would purposely plan runs that included these hills. When you see a hill, you can see the top. You can see the end destination. I would look at the top, visualize myself there, then put my head down and focus on the road and each step I was taking. I would just grind away at that hill until I hit the top. That was my "in the moment" challenge, and that hill had to be conquered!

- Running downhill. The good news about running up the hill is that you then get to run down, but running downhill is not as easy as it sounds. If you do not practice it, you can overstep and injure yourself. It is simply a different type of running; a different set of muscles are used, and they can be very sore afterwards. I could not miss out on this different type of exercise, so I had to incorporate it into my training plans.

- During my longer runs, I would be in running mode for a minimum of an hour. Since I ran so much and for so long, I would spend a lot of time alone with myself. Over a long run, as I'm physically going through multiple stages of bliss and pain, I also go through multiple stages of emotions—and boy, do I have lots of emotions. I realized that this is normal, and I used these emotions to get me through the run and to the end.

- I learned to incorporate a few different mantras and affirmations when I run. Things like: "You got this," and "You can't stop yet." One that got me through some of my long races was: "One step at time." I was able to focus my mind on each step. Every step forward was closer to the finish. Instead of being overwhelmed with the overall race, I spent time focusing only on that next step, then the next step.

- Each and every run was a success, and I made sure to acknowledge that. The run may have been a hard one.

I may have felt crappy, been very slow, or even walked some of it. I may not have gone as far as I wanted to go, but none of those things matter. The fact that I showed up, got out of bed, walked out the door, and did my run was a massive success.

- I purposefully vary my runs. I run different distances every day, I never run the same route, and I switch between road and trail. This keeps me interested and motivated to keep going.

- I realized early on that there are good and bad techniques when you run. What is my cadence? Length of stride? Posture? I had to find the most efficient form and style of running for me. This took practice and research. There us a lot of information out there about running, and I used it to find what works best for me.

- If you want to be a runner, then you have to run. When you stop running for a period of time, it takes some time to get your mind and body back into being able to run again. This is true for anything you want to do.

- My running routes would sometimes be a path directly away from my starting point. I would run as far as I felt good. This then required me to turn around and run the same distance back; I had no choice. This ensured that I got the proper training and miles in, and it also kept me challenged. It did not allow me to quit.

PUPPY RUNS

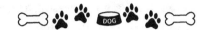

Have you ever watched a puppy run? They are not very good at it. They fall down a lot, and Duder was no exception. We brought him home to us when he was about eight weeks old. Up to this point, he had been learning to walk and had started to learn to run. So, at eight weeks, he had already been practicing and getting better. Soon after, he grew bigger and stronger. He soon became very good at running.

Got me thinking...

Do you want to give running a try? Every new skill starts from nothing, and it helps to practice the basics at first. So, this chapter will be my running starter kit. Here are some of the things I learned in my running journey that would be helpful for you to consider.

Let's start with the Three Ms.

Mind

Why do you want to run? Running is hard and you better have a good reason to do it. If your reason why is to lose weight, then that is a bad reason. I would not recommend running as a mechanism for losing weight. I did not start running until I had lost most of my weight, I was walking and hiking. Running can be physical hard on your body, certainly hard on knees, and legs in general. If you are overweight, then it is that much harder and potentially damaging.

So, you need to find good reasons why. Maybe you want to run a marathon and check that off the bucket list? You have friends that run, and they want you to run with them? You have seen runners and you just want to give it a try? Do you want to win a race? At a minimum, you need to determine some reason why you want to do this.

Meal

Running is one of the more caloric burning exercises you can do. Your body burns a great deal of fuel when you run, and there are different variations of running that will burn more calories. The type of fuel you take in makes a difference as well. What I have learned is that there is not one single path to follow. There are so many ideas and opinions out there, and everybody will respond to fueling plans differently.

Let me give you an example from my own experience. I had an ultramarathon coming up: an extremely vigorous fifty-mile trail race. I had my running plan in place, and

I had a fueling plan. I followed a traditional very high carb diet for runners. I was putting in many training miles each week. During this training period, I stopped weighing myself on the scale. One week before the race, I had pulled a muscle in my right leg and decided that I was not able to run the race. I was disappointed, but I believe my body was telling me that I was not prepared to do that race. The next disappointment happened after I got back on the scale. During that training phase, I had gained twenty pounds. Even with all the running and training I was doing, and even with the mostly clean fueling plan, I was adding body fat.

There is a saying out there that states, "You cannot outrun a diet." This is true. I have since moved my fueling to a low carb plan. This also helps my brain. The bottom line is that if you want to run, you need to a fueling plan that works for you.

Move

Now we can get started. So, should you just walk out the door and start running? This might work for some of you, but if you are new to it, here is where I would start.

Take a week, seven days, and walk for thirty minutes every day. Find the time of day that works and start the habit of going out to do it. After seven days, start to add some running into your walking routine. Keep going out every day and walk/run until you are running more than walking.

Having the correct running gear is also important to start running. Shoes and socks are important, and quality running shoes and socks are also expensive. Before you take the plunge into all the best gear, I would explore your "why." Give yourself a few weeks of daily walking and short runs to first make sure this is something worth pursuing. If it is, then you need to get quality gear. When shoe store salespeople see me walk in, they try to hide. I am a pain in the butt as a customer. If I need a new pair of shoes, I will try on almost everything they have, narrow it down to top three or four choices, then narrow those down to the one pair that feels and works the best for my feet. I am running around in the store on all these different shoes. This can be a one-to-two-hour process. Gear is important.

After deciding to fully dedicate yourself to getting into running, you will need to grow and develop into a runner. I believe there are three phases of running growth. The first is your lungs and heart. When you start running, you will run out of breath and your heart rate will be cranking fast. Eventually you will find a pace where you can control your breathing, not run out of breath, and keep your heart rate healthy.

The second phase is your legs and muscles. As with anything, when you use those leg muscles on a regular basis, they will get stronger and more able to sustain longer runs. I remember after my first time running five miles, I was sore for three days. After my first half marathon, I could hardly walk for a week. I now run ten to fifteen miles every weekend with no soreness. Your muscles will get stronger.

The third and final phase is your mind. When you start running for longer periods of time, your lungs and heart should be in a good, steady place. Your legs and muscles will be able to do it, but your mind will then become the thing that is telling you to stop. This is where your true grit comes out, and you will be turning back to your "why." You will ask yourself, "Why the hell am I doing this?" If you don't have a good answer, then you will not be able to go on.

Running has brought a great deal of satisfaction to my life, and I plan on running as long as my body can do it. When it can't, I will find something different.

MOMENTS OF BLISS

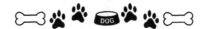

Duder and I love to go out on trail runs. Our runs vary from shorter (two to five miles) to longer (five to ten miles).

When we would do a longer run, I'd always notice how Duder would change his patterns during our runs. I'd also notice how I would change my patterns and how I felt over the long run.

When we would start, Duder would be in crazy mode: running around, sniffing everything, peeing on every leaf he could find, not at all focused on the run. One of the trails we would go on was quite hilly with lots of climbing, sometimes with over 1,000 vertical feet. On the way down from the climb, there was one downhill stretch that was one of my favorites. It's a single-track trail that's packed with grass and flowers and lined with trees on both sides, and it has a small creek running next to it. Sometimes it felt like running in a tunnel. During the long runs, we would be at mile seven or eight at this point. Duder would be in his zone. He was not peeing everywhere; he was not sniffing everything; he was not running off the trail. He had a nice, even pace, running right in front of me. You could see he was very focused and enjoying the moment.

Got me thinking...

Watching Duder on this stretch allowed me to absorb what I was experiencing as well. I had been running hard, up and down for over an hour. Heading down this perfect little stretch of trail, I would stop my audiobook or podcast and "run naked." This is a term used in the running community that refers to running without any headphones, GPS, or any other technology.

In this moment, my legs were cruising and felt good. I could hear only the sounds of nature. I could also hear the rhythmic sound of my steps as I glided down the trail. The term "runner's high" comes to mind.

In these moments of bliss, the world was gone. That never-ending to-do list did not matter. Those emails did not matter. The stress and anxiety did not exist. Those annoying parts of life were just gone. It truly felt like I was floating through time and space—just a guy and his dog, together, living in the moment.

I make sure I take the time to appreciate these moments. They are invaluable.

This really got me thinking...

How can I make these moments happen in other places in my life?

Let's take the example of running naked (no

headphones, GPS, etc.). To be present and find your moments of bliss, you need to go naked with what you do.

When you spend time with your spouse or partner, your family, your kids, or your grandkids, is that phone and smart watch distracting you? Is that TV on? If they are, you are not living in the moment.

When the Blonde and I go somewhere together, a date out to eat for example, the phone is put away or turned off. I purposefully make extreme effort to offer all of my attention to her. She sees this behavior and then does the same back to me. These are the times when, together, you can find those moments of bliss.

THE TRAIL LIFE

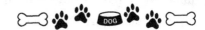

As you are now very much aware, Duder and I love the trails. The ideas for this book became real for me while out on the trails.

Got me thinking...

At one point in this process, I started a blog to capture these ideas I had. I then stopped the blog and started to collect these ideas into this book.

What I realized was that when the blog started, I started looking for ideas to write about. Every time Duder and I would go out hiking or running, I was unconsciously looking for ideas.

My mind was in a state of active idea generation. It was open and ready to collect any ideas and information in for processing. This state of mind, I refer to as a growth mindset. I was consciously and unconsciously wanting to grow. I wanted ideas, information, and knowledge. I wanted to incorporate them into my life.

When you open yourself up to new ideas and bring

them in, your mind expands and starts working in different ways. You get used to new thoughts and your mind will adjust. I now crave information. My mind is always looking and searching.

This can be applied to anything. When you open your mind and put it in search mode, it will find it.

SITUATIONAL MOTIVATION

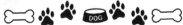

Duder and Roxie seem to be constantly on alert for noises. Roxie is the more obnoxious one. She will hear a noise outside and burst into full barking mode and run outside to catch whatever she heard. Duder will sometimes follow suit, jumping up and running outside with her. Sometimes, if he is sitting comfy on the couch, he will not follow and simply stay where he is.

Got me thinking...

We have all been motivated by a deadline. Motivated by events. Motivated by what people around us are doing. We are motivated by the current situation.

I was motivated to continue my transformation journey. I was motivated to keep growing. The key is how to convert this situational motivation to discipline. How do I find the discipline to continue executing the changes I've made to my life? How do I stay on track?

Finding the discipline to continue doing things you

know you should do is the hard part. You might feel motivated, but that does not always equate or convert to the actual doing.

When I need to find my motivation, I will revisit my "why." I have identified specific reasons why I want to continue going down that path. My "why" feeds my purpose and discipline.

Here are some other techniques I use:

- I ask my future self what he would do.
- Ask myself why I wouldn't do it, and how will my day be impacted from neglecting that responsibility.
- Conversely, ask myself how my day would be affected if I *did* do it.

Many times, to add a sense of accountability, I will ask these questions while looking at myself in the mirror.

TAKING THE DOGS WITH ME

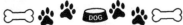

As my running journey expanded to longer and endurance running, I could not always take the dogs with me on my longer runs. They did not like this at all. They wanted to go, be with me, be a part of the run.

Got me thinking...

Throughout my day, there were times when I would take my wedding ring off. When I would exercise, do yard work, or even shower, the ring would come off.

But, when I'd go out on a run, I became adamant that I had to put my wedding ring on. This was my way of taking the Blonde with me. She is not a runner and does not run with me, so this allowed me to keep her with me. Five years ago, when I started on this new journey, I needed her with me for all of it, not just the running. This journey is truly just as much hers as it is mine.

We do our best to plan and talk about our future, what is important to us, and what things we should do. We are in this together. I did not go out and do this on my own; she has been with me through it all. She will admit that it is not always easy though. She has started getting herself out of her own comfort zone and doing new things as well. One accomplishment that has come from it is becoming a certified yoga instructor.

Essentially, this book and the transformation it recounts is *our* tale, not just mine.

RUNNING ON THE ROAD

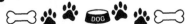

When I take the dogs on the road, they have to be on their leashes. I use a hip belt, which is a loop that goes around my waist, where I can then connect a split leash that is attached to the dogs. This allows me to keep my hands free as I run but won't let the dogs stray too far. The split leash keeps the two dogs together. They had to learn how to run next to each other and even anticipate each other's movements. Sometimes Roxie will want to go one way and try to drag Duder along. Sometimes, Duder will stop to pee or poop and Roxie does not want to stop. She will try to keep going and drag him along. Sometimes they run in perfect harmony and in unison.

They ultimately have the same destination, and since they are attached, they will get there together.

Got me thinking...

While watching Duder and Roxie in this scenario, I'd wonder about my relationship with the Blonde. Here we are, going along in life, attached together by a choice that we both made to be together. That choice is our split leash. We are legally married, but that legal binding can be dissolved. So, what ultimately keeps us together is a mutual choice.

Sometimes, one of us will try to go one way, but the other does not want to. We will drag each other around, pulling, pushing, stopping, just like Duder and Roxie.

There were times when we did not have the same destination in mind. This caused a lot of tension on that leash keeping us together. Sometimes it would get stretched pretty dang tight.

When we began truly talking about our future, where we wanted to go, what our together destination is, that leash became a good thing. Less pulling on each other, less one going a different direction without the other. We were working together. Moving forward in unison.

DUDER LOOKS FOR SIGNALS

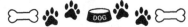

When I need to go somewhere, let's say to the store or a hike, I will get up and gather my keys, wallet, water bottle, and whatever else I might need for my mini adventure. Duder has gotten very good at watching for these actions from me. He believes that he is going with me every time. This always gets him excited. He doesn't know where we are going, I think he just wants to be with me, and he knows that these are good times to do that.

Sometimes he will see these signals and "sneak" over towards to the door. I am not kidding—he will literally tiptoe across the hardwood floor. Normally you would hear his toenails on the floor, but when he does this, you cannot. He will stand by the door, ready to go. He is sneaking because he does not want Roxie to go. Just him. Just the two of us. He wants me all to himself.

He is excited. We will get outside, and he is jumping all around and just plain happy to be going somewhere with me.

When I observe this, it always makes me smile. These

are the simple things that keep us sane.

Got me thinking...

In my relationship with the Blonde, she wants me to go with her on these shopping trips or to run errands. What if I responded to her the same way that Duder responds to me? Pure excited to be with her and go to the grocery store! Might sound sarcastic, but actually showing her that I want to be with her makes some dramatic differences.

This is true with your kids, other family members, and even your close friends. Be excited to be with them, show them that you are excited to be with them. You do this by focusing your attention on them, asking them about their life—and most importantly, put your stupid phone away.

DUDER DREAMS

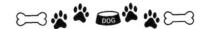

Sometimes when Duder sleeps, you can see that he is dreaming. His breathing starts to get faster, his legs move, and it appears almost like he is chasing an animal. I assume he is in his happy place, chasing rabbits out on the trail, but I have no way of knowing for sure.

Got me thinking...

What do my dreams mean?

I started to keep a pad of paper and pen next to my bed. On those occasions when I would wake up from a dream and have a vivid memory of it, I'd take a moment and write the basics down. This helped me remember the dream later in the day.

I do not know what dreams mean. I do not know what is going on in my mind during that night to have that particular dream. What I do know is that, sometimes, my dreams play a role in my perspective. I can interpret them and get what I need out of them.

One night, I had a dream that I was crouched over a pot

of red-hot molten steel. I was trying to reach something on the other side. It was hot. I was losing my strength. I could not reach the item. I tried to stand back up, but I did not have the strength. I was getting closer to the hot metal. It was starting to burn. I had to get back up. I pushed with my last bit of determination and strength. I had to get away from the heat! I had to stand up!!

Then I woke up. I wrote this scene down.

I took the liberty of interpreting this dream. I am fifty-five years old. I am getting closer to the molten heat. If I do not stand up, if I do not put in every ounce of energy and determination to get away from the heat, then all will be lost.

For me, the heat represented my past actions and life perspective. Standing up represented doing something different. Stop going back to my old habits, my old thinking, and my old self-talk.

My determination to do different things was embedded deep and affecting my dreams.

WHAT IS ROXIE THINKING ABOUT?

I was in my office at my desk, I looked over at Roxie, who was lying on her bed in the corner. She had this strange and zoned out look on her face. Maybe she was just tired, but it always makes me wonder what is going on in her head. What are the thoughts that dogs have? Do they even have thoughts? Are they self-aware?

Got me thinking...

We all spend most of our days in our own minds. Conversations with ourselves, opinions about the world, what to eat, how we feel about ourselves, and how we feel about life. How many thousands of thoughts do we have in a day? It is a little crazy to think about.

Just because they are common and frequent, it doesn't mean that these thoughts and talks with yourself are always beneficial. Sometimes, they can be detrimental to your health. Some people really struggle with this, so they turn to things, such as drugs or alcohol, that help them escape from this world. There are other methods to control the chaos in your mind that might exist.

With my transformation, I have purposefully turned off the TV, reduced phone use, and generally tried to reduce the inputs into my life. I now spend more time with myself, in my own mind and in my own thoughts. For me, running or doing anything involving movement are the best times with myself.

One thing I did was embrace the idea of mantras. These are statements that I used daily to keep myself on track. They worked for me. When I would have an idea or someone was talking about it in a book or podcast, I would write them down on my whiteboard. At one point, I made a list of important statements. I printed it out and made three copies; one is next to my bed, one is in my office, and I keep the last one in my wallet. I read them out loud every morning and every night. Here is my list:

- You got this.
- How bad do I want it?
- I am willing.
- I am a badass.
- Always move forward, one step at a time.
- I am relentless.
- I am not willing to sacrifice my future self.
- I don't want to die.
- I don't care what the world thinks.
- I am not going back.

- I am worthy.
- I show my gratitude for life in all that I do.
- I am willing to do the work to bring wealth into my life.
- I am excited to bring the power of dogs to the world.
- I am proud of myself.
- AM: What are my intentions?
- PM: What went well today?

I would say that the Blonde has a more chaotic mind than I do. It is much harder for her to calm the thoughts and clear the mind. It takes work and intentional planning to do this. She discovered yoga. After time and a great deal of practice, the Blonde has found a way to use yoga to help calm the chaos in her mind. She even became a yoga instructor to teach others how to do the same. I have done yoga with the Blonde and have experienced the benefits for myself.

Running calms my mind now, but this only came from practice and dedication. While I'm running, I can focus my thoughts, contemplate ideas, meditate, envision the future, and effectively clear out anything that causes strife within myself.

DUDER'S CHALLENGE

What do you currently do to calm your mind? If you don't have an effective method, figure out what works for you. Take time to focus on yourself and on your thoughts. Meditate. Walk. Breathe. Try something new that you think might help.

ADDING SOME DISTANCE

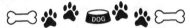

There were many times when Duder and I were out hiking or running on the trails, and he would smell something off the trail and spend some time investigating. He would never just ignore it. I would keep hiking, and he would stay back to continue his investigation. No matter how far away I would get—and sometimes it got to be quite a bit of distance—he'd always come back to me. It seemed like he always kept track of where I was.

Got me thinking...

I want to tell you a story about my oldest daughter. When she hit thirteen or fourteen, things started to change for her. She was hanging out with the wrong crowd and got involved with things that were not good for her. She was going down a very bad path. Over time, she started to get into trouble with the law and started getting into drugs.

As a parent, my first reaction was that I needed to save her. We need to do everything we can to "fix" her. What should we do? Why won't she listen to us? I'm her dad.

She's my oldest daughter. What did I do wrong? Did I not do enough? All of these thoughts and questions haunted me.

There were times when we had no idea where she was, and other times where we knew where she was—because she'd be in jail. There were some long nights that caused the Blonde and I considerable anguish. Sometimes it truly shut me down.

What I realized was that I needed to distance myself from her. The only thing I could do was keep track of her and provide her with love. This was her life and these were her choices, so she needed to get herself out of the place she was in. No one else was going to do that for her.

This distancing exercise included some hard choices for me and the Blonde, including that we would no longer offer financial support, nor would we bail her out of jail. She had to learn how to make it without us taking care of her mistakes.

During these tumultuous times, she had a couple of kids, and her children were affected by her choices as well. It was to the point that she could not care for them.

She eventually found her way out. She essentially hit bottom, spent some time in jail, got out, and made the choice to do something different. She found work doing concrete cutting. She started listening to self-improvement podcasts while she worked. She began to own the choices she made. She got herself clean. She found herself a good job. She began to make good choices that had a good impact both on her own life and on her two kids. She is now influencing others and making her own impact on the world.

This applies to my transformation as well. I needed to change, and it was my own decision to make that change and put in the work for it. No matter how much the Blonde wanted to change me, she could not do it for me. She had to distance herself from me, and I had to make the decision.

JUST MOVE ON

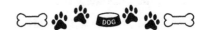

"If it's not going to matter in five years, do not spend more than five minutes being upset by it." —Ed Mylett

When Duder was a puppy, we went through the phase of training and teaching proper behaviors. We needed to train him not to pee in the house, or chew on the Blonde's couch, or hump my leg. Since there are so many different ways to train a dog to do certain things, we had to discover what worked with all of us.

During this phase, Duder would do something that he was not supposed to do, which would get him into trouble. He would be scolded, and he understood that he did something wrong and that we were not happy about it. Over time, he learned not to do those things.

We also incorporated the positive aspect by rewarding him with attention, and occasionally treats, for good behaviors.

One thing I noticed was that if he ever got scolded, he truly did understand. He would put his tail down between his legs for a period of time, but it did not last long. He easily got over it and was always back to his happy, tail-wagging self.

Got me thinking...

Do we have the same ability to move on from things that happen to us? There are always events and other aspects of our lives that might cause us to put our tails between our legs. How do we move on?

These events might be small, or they might be big and catastrophic. Regardless of the proportion of it, most of us have had a past interaction with someone that we cannot move on from. The thought of them or the interaction gnaws at us, no matter how much time passes. This is actually quite silly if you think about it; that memory and those thoughts are in control of us.

There are many techniques out there to help you move on. These might include talking to the person about it, talking to someone else about it, or writing it down (so you can get it out of your head).

The first step is to become aware that these thoughts are causing a problem, then finding some techniques to move on.

I think of Duder and his example helps me.

TRUST

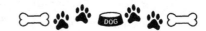

When we go hiking, we like to go to new places, hike new trails, and go on new adventures. Wherever we go, Duder will always go with me. He follows me wherever I take him. He trusts that I will not lead him astray.

Got me thinking...

One thing the Blonde and I like to do is hop on my motorcycle and go for rides. I drive and she rides on the back. Riding fast on two wheels can be scary sometimes. The Blonde has more guts than I do; she is putting all her trust in me as I drive and navigate this thing with all the other cars and traffic.

Trusting people is risky. I think we have all been burned by someone at some point in our lives. It will always make us weary.

The Blonde and I have been together for a very long time. Over the years, things have not always been good, and we have had some very rocky times. There have been occasions where that trust that we should have in one another has been broken (mostly by me). These are the toughest times to overcome. Trust in each other must be restored before truly recovering.

I had to take some time and contemplate the trust between the Blonde and me. At fifty years old, it was not great. I started with myself. Am I giving her reasons to not trust me? The answer might come as a quick "No," but there are other questions that factor into this one. Do I hide things from my partner? Do I lie to them?

It's so easy to get focused on your partner and what they are doing. But stop and worry about your side first. Do you want to have trust in your relationship? Then don't do things that break that trust, and don't give them any reason not to trust you.

Here's the first test to try. Does your partner know the PIN to access your phone, and if not, would you give it to them? In the past, I would not have given the Blonde my phone. Now, she knows my PIN and can access my phone anytime. This led to her sharing the same information with me—so it goes both ways. This simple act of trust between us goes a LONG way. This was me taking steps to build back the trust that had been lost over time.

DUDER'S VIEW OF THE WORLD

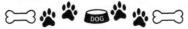

"Each person does see the world in a different way. There is not a single unifying, objective truth. We're all limited by our perspective."
—Siri Hustvedt

Duder is pretty short compared to me—most dogs are. His literal view of the world is from a much lower perspective. He must look up when he wants to see me.

One day when we were hiking along a trail that was lined with some bushes, grass, and trees, I noticed that his view of the trail was different than mine. I got down on all fours and started crawling along the trail. I wanted to see what the trail looked like from his view. It was very different. The bushes were much taller, the grass was in my face. I liked it better down there, but my knees were getting scraped up, so I had to stop crawling. Also, the other hikers were looking at me funny.

Got me thinking...

Every person on this planet has a different view, which I refer to as our inner perspective, or IP. So many factors play a role in that perspective and in our opinion of our existence.

When I think back to my old self, my IP was very different than it is today. I have changed so much about my life and have so many more inputs, knowledge, and information coming in.

One thing that has changed drastically is my opinion of the world and the role that I play in it. Life is what I make it. Life is how I choose to perceive it. I can choose to be cynical and negative, or I can choose to be hopeful and grateful. It truly is a choice we make.

I have also chosen to enhance my IP with different inputs than I have in the past. Everything you do, read, watch, and listen to and all of the people you interact with impact your IP. You can be in the exact same circumstances, but your perspective is different.

STOP AND BREATHE

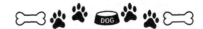

When Duder and I would head out for a hike, we'd hop in the truck—me in the driver's seat and Duder in the back seat. I would open the back window and he would always stick his head out. On occasion, he would close his eyes, point his head up at the blue sky, and soak in the sun. When he'd do this, he seemed very relaxed, like he was living in the moment.

Got me thinking...

In our busy lives, how often do we neglect ourselves? Do we take the time to breathe? Do we stop and look up at the blue sky? Do we live in the moment?

It is very easy to let the anxiety, rush, and toils of life overtake us. When this happens, it usually causes more anxiety and stress.

There are moments of overwhelming and immediate anxiety within people's lives. These are times when we should stop and breathe. It might be as simple as stopping what you are doing, closing your eyes, breathing deep for five big breaths, then reevaluating the situation.

There are also times when we get too busy and are so focused on the task at hand that we miss living our lives. It is important to appreciate the little things in life. It's the cliché of stopping to smell the flowers, and it really does help. This is an exercise you can use and incorporate at any time during the day.

So, learn from Duder. Sometimes, you just need to stop and breathe.

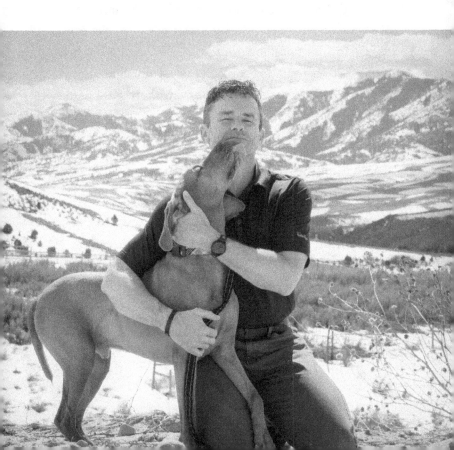

QUIT BARKING!!

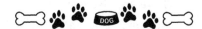

I had Duder and Roxie out for a run the other day. We were on a road run because the trails were wet from a rainstorm. I had them on the split leash and hip belt while we were running through our local neighborhood of houses and a park. Along the way, there were some houses where other dogs lived. When we passed them, the other dogs would run up to fence they were in, start barking, and basically cause a commotion. At the same time, Duder and Roxie would respond with their own barking and try to pull me to the fence. Two dogs on one leash yanking on you is not fun.

When these other dogs would start barking at us, I remember getting annoyed at them. Why don't their owners train them better? What is wrong with them? I wish they would stop. Then I realized that my dogs were not behaving any better. Why was I so annoyed at the other ones?

Got me thinking...

I used to view the world and people around me as those other dogs. Barking at me and annoying me. It was always them. They were the problem. They were the reason for my feelings. During my transformation, I had to change that mindset.

Maybe I should think about my role in everything first: What am I doing or adding to a situation? What am I not doing, and what didn't I do? Am I the one barking? This reversal of thought helped me recognize my own actions in any given situation, which has helped me understand how to own my actions. Doing this is a key part of making change. It takes effort and time to change those thought patterns.

As I was evaluating my relationship with the Blonde, this pattern effectively saved our relationship. It is so easy to blame her and get mad at her. Why did she say that? Why did she do that? I would always believe that she was the cause of strife between us.

I started an exercise in my head. If the Blonde and I were engaged in something together and she did or said anything that would trigger me, I'd pause and ask myself: What is my role in this? Is there something I did? What should I do now? I had to start with me—with my side of things—and own my reaction. It takes courage to do this.

But first, make sure you train your own dogs.

DUDER AND THE MOOSE

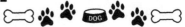

Duder and I were hiking on a trail in Utah called Mount Timpanogos. It is the second highest peak in Utah and is an elevation of 11,752 ft. It can be a challenging hike and climb.

About halfway up the trail, we were on a single track with lots of grass and trees around us. Duder was running ahead of me off the leash. He was around a corner and out of my sight. Then, suddenly, he came back around the corner, running as fast as he could—I mean, he was cruising!! He went right by me and kept going. I just stopped, standing there a little flabbergasted. What they heck was going on? I walked slowly up the trail and looked around the corner. Ahead was a very large moose standing next to what I assumed to be her baby moose. Duder must have tried to say hello, but that mama moose was not having any of that. Any mother in nature can be dangerous and must be treated with caution. This moose must have scared the crap out of Duder, and that is why he went running away.

Got me thinking...

This mama moose would do anything to protect her young. Would I do the same for my kids? What am I doing for my kids now? What will I provide for them in the future? How will I continue to provide for them after I'm gone? What is my legacy with my kids? How will they remember me?

I had to truly take some time to ponder these questions. What did they learn from me? What aspects of my life were embedded in their minds and their lives?

All three of my daughters are out in the world, living their own lives now. They are all doing different things. They are making their own way in this world.

I truly want to be a great dad. There were times in my life when I know I wasn't great. I can spend all the time in the world with regrets and pity parties, but it doesn't matter. What matters is now. Throughout my transformation, this concept hit home to me in so many ways. All I can do is be a great dad right now and every day going forward.

This now applies to me as a grandpa, or as one of my grandkids calls me, BeeBop. Grandkids are the best, so I want to inspire mine. I want to be part of their lives. I want them to be equipped to find their own way in this world. I joke with my kids that the only reason I had them was to give me grandkids.

How do you be a good dad or grandpa? Teach by example. Teach them to do hard things. Teach basic things in life. Teach them how to live and survive in this world on their own. They have to learn to find their own way. Don't carry them; make them carry themselves. At the same time, be reliable. Let your children know that they can fall back on you as they're growing and learning, and set them straight when they waver.

As a parent, you will have an impact on your kids regardless of the role you have in their lives. Everything you do will leave an impression on your kids; it may be something you are not even aware of. So be conscious of your actions as a parent. Do everything you can to be a positive influence. Be the best parent you can be.

MIND GAMES

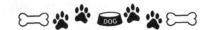

The Blonde and I like to play a game with our dogs. We call it "Find It." We have a particular red chew toy that we use. As soon as we pick it up, the dogs know that we're about to play the game. We take the dogs to another room and tell them to stay, which they do. I then hide the chew toy somewhere in the house, go back to the dogs, and tell them to "find it." They proceed to run around and search for the red toy. Sometimes it's easy for them, and sometimes it takes a while. But it's a great exercise for them to practice the use of their minds.

Got me thinking...

Over the last few years, I have embraced the idea of learning. I started to read on a regular basis, listened to books and podcasts, and generally tried to soak up new ideas and thoughts. I was always searching for new information. I am always looking for my red bone.

There were periods of time where I would get relaxed in my learning, when my discipline would slip. I would not read my book for a week. I would start listening to music instead of podcasts. It took some time to see the result of this, but it affected my motivation towards my eating habits, my training habits, my work habits—all of it. There is a strong connection between exercising the mind and exercising the body, and being disciplined is critical.

There are other ways to exercise the mind, such as meditation. Turn off the TV or mindless shows. Stay off social media. Stop watching or reading the news.

DUDER'S CHALLENGE

Stop watching TV for a week. Seven days. Find something else to do and see how it impacts you.

TRIGGERS

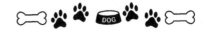

During some downtime over one of the holiday seasons, I sat down and did a rewatch of one of my favorite movie series: *The Lord of the Rings* trilogy. Duder was sitting next to me, lounging like he likes to do. Nothing else about the movie startled him, except when the character Gollum started talking. He quickly jumped up and started growling at the screen. What was it about Gollum that triggered him?

Got me thinking...

Do we have Gollums in our lives? Are there things or people that just bother us, maybe without reason? Things that make us jump up and growl?

As an example, there's this traffic light that's close to my house. When I'm driving, that thing is red every time. For some reason, it bothers me. It causes a reaction in my mind and body—nothing too dramatic, but it is there. When this feeling comes in, my response to everything else around me changes. If I am sitting at that light, getting irked, and someone pulls too close behind me, I react to that person. If a cloud blocks the sun, I react to the weather. A song that I do not like comes on the radio, I react to the station. So on and so on. I realize that I'm in a "state of reaction" all because of that stupid red light. I have no control over that light. I cannot make it go green. So why does that object have control over me?

Why? Because I let it in my mind and my thoughts. I choose to let it define how I feel at the moment. If I take a step back from this scenario, it's kind of funny. There's no logical reason why this traffic light should control me.

I had to learn some new tricks when the "Gollum reflex" started to kick in. I stopped and did some self-talk. "I am in control." "I will not let that thing control me."

In the case of Duder, he would growl at Gollum, then he would stop and go back to his lounging ways. Do the same.

IS DUDER HAPPY?

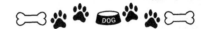

Duder wags his tail all the time, and mostly, it's because he's happy. When he's excited, it can be a little dangerous. It's like a weapon—you need to stay clear of that thing.

There are some very simple things that will make him happy. When he gets a good treat from me, he is happy. When he knows we are heading out for a walk, he gets happy. When he can sit down next to me, he is happy.

Got me thinking...

What are the signs that we, as humans, are happy? Do we have an internal definition for happiness? How do we know when we are happy?

I have spent a great deal of time over the last few years evaluating my happiness and trying to define what the word means to me. I have read books, listened to podcasts, meditated on the subject, and talked to people about it as well. I now believe that a huge part of happiness is a choice. We must make the choice to be happy. This is not an easy thing to do, but it is critical to try and incorporate.

There are some common society beliefs out there: If I make more money, I will be happy. If I get into a relationship, I will be happy. If I get that new car, I will be happy.

When we see rich people, we assume they are happy. When we see married people, we assume they are happy. When someone is driving that cool car we want, we assume they are happy.

Our happiness cannot be conditional. If we plant the seed in our minds that we make more money, we'll be happy, then we also set up the condition that we cannot be happy UNTIL we make more money. This is not a good belief to have.

The Blonde and I recently did an exercise of defining what our goals and aspirations are in our lives. We started tossing around ideas and writing them down. Then we organized them by priority and identified which goals would lead to the achievement of others.

We discovered that the highest level of goals and aspirations for us was "Happiness and Wellbeing." We simply wanted to be together and be happy. Well, we decided that we were going to be happy. We decided to view life with that goal in mind. Being thankful for the small things and embedding that gratitude in your thoughts will get you to that state of happiness.

I do know that now that I think better, eat better, relationship better, exercise better, and have better inputs, I am happy. I finally have a path, I have direction, and I have hope. For me, this equates to happiness.

One thing I do know: Duder makes me happy.

HEADING DOWN THE WRONG TRAIL

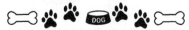

When Duder and I go hiking, we have access to an open area with hills and several different trails of varying difficulty. I try to take different trails, depending on time, weather, and how I feel. This is a great area because it allows Duder to go off leash and get in the running that the Vizsla breed desperately needs.

We drive over and have a few different spots where we can park. When we stop, I open the door and Duder bolts out, taking off down one of the trails with great excitement. He doesn't even know which trail I'm going to take. I then begin my hike and head down a different trail. Duder is always aware and monitors my location. He will stop, see that I am going a different direction, then run back towards me with even more energy than before. He does not mope. He does not whine. He does not complain. He does not get mad that I am going a different direction.

Got me thinking...

Our life is full of many different trails and paths we can take. We do not always take the one that's best for us. Think about some of the wrong directions you have gone in your life. We all have them. The key to this is how do we respond.

I can recall a particular business venture I began many years ago. Sometime after starting, it became obvious that it was a wrong trail. At the time, my ego kicked in and I had a hard time stopping and turning around. I can see myself pausing, taking a deep breath, shoulders slouched, head hanging low in depression while trying to decide where to go. If I had followed Duder's example, I would have realized I was on the wrong path and began the immediate journey back to a different path with renewed excitement and energy.

DUDER'S CHALLENGE

What are some examples in your life where you went down the wrong path? Maybe in a relationship, with your health, or with your spirituality. Try to identify times in your life where you had to turn around and backtrack after realizing you were going in a bad direction.

Now, look at where you are now and see if you are currently on a wrong path. If you are, stop, find out where you want to be—which path you would like to be on instead—turn around, and head towards that different trail with your head held high. Appreciate anything you've learned from going this direction and be excited to be moving forward (because you are—moving forward—despite having to go back from where you came).

THE PEE INTERRUPTION

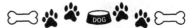

I was out on an early morning run the other day. I had Duder and Roxie with me. We were out on the road, they were on the split leash, and I had the waist leash on with these two running up in front of me. When we do this kind of run, we run through neighborhoods, typically on the sidewalks.

It is normal for the two of them to stop and either pee or poop on the run at some point, however, on this particular run, Duder was in full "pee mode." We were out about forty-five minutes, and he stopped to pee twenty-one times. Anyone who has ever done any running knows how annoying it is to have to stop this often. When you get going, you get into the groove with fluid motion. It's one thing when you're in full stride and you have to slow down, but Duder stops on a dime to put out that leg and drop that tinkle of pee on a little bush. This makes me almost trip over him, and one time, he even knocked me to the ground.

Duder's bladder cannot be that big—he can only hold so much pee in there. But after a while, when there was no more pee, he still had to stop, lift his leg, and go through the motions of peeing. I can't make him stop.

Got me thinking...

While going through my transformation, there were many times I felt like I was on a run; I was in a groove with good forward momentum. I was incorporating all of these ideas and lessons into my thinking and doing. I had projects I was working on. I was writing this book. I was working on myself steadily.

What I have discovered is that there will always be things that make the process stop. Just like Duder will interrupt a run and make me stop on a dime, life happens and knocks you out of your groove. Life tries to make you stop. There can be things or events that are out of our control that bring us to a halt. However, I would argue that most times, these things are in our control, and we choose to let them stop us.

Spend too much time on your phone, watching TV, or couch sitting? Why did you eat that, even though you know it is not good for you? Did you do something to harm your relationship? These are things that seemed to stop me in my tracks; they stopped me from moving forward as I wanted to do. Still, after every mishap, bad decision, and life circumstance, I eventually started moving again.

So, even though Duder has to stop all the frickin time,

it doesn't mean my run is over—I don't turn around and go home. We keep moving forward. The intent is to keep going down the path, no matter how many times we stop.

This is true for our life journey. Life happens and interrupts, but the journey will continue. The interruptions are only pit stops on the way to the finish.

WHERE TO PEE?

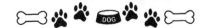

Duder seems to be somewhat particular about where he pees. He has to find that perfect spot—usually somewhere on a tree, bush, or rock. After he finds that perfect spot and takes care of his business, he struts around a bit; he is very proud of himself.

Roxie seems to stop and pee wherever and whenever she needs to. She understands that peeing in the house is not okay, but outside, anything goes.

Got me thinking...

The Blonde is more like Duder in this scenario. She is very particular about where she goes to the bathroom.

However, on one occasion, we were out running errands together. She had to pee. We were on our way to Walmart and still had some time before we got there. She was doing the potty dance in the car, ready to burst. We pulled up in front of Walmart, and she hopped out of the car and ran in. I then parked the car, took my time, and walked in. I headed over to the restrooms and went in as well.

I made my way to one of the urinals and there was another guy there. He was having a conversation with someone, or so it seemed, but no one else was in sight.

I then heard the Blonde's voice from the stall next to the urinals. The guy was talking to my wife in the men's room. She was in such a hurry that she had run into the men's room to pee. At that moment, I was not sure how to respond, but it did put a smile on my face. I ended up telling the other guy that it was my wife he was talking to.

After some initial embarrassment, we had a pleasant time for the rest of our visit at Walmart.

DUDER, FINISH THE POOP!

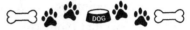

Duder, Roxie, and I were out on a walk the other day. We started walking down a trail. Duder began sniffing around, spinning in circles. I knew what was coming. He found his spot and began his routine of taking a dump. As I was observing this activity, Roxie went running by Duder. Duder stopped mid-poop and just had to follow Roxie. He ran about twenty yards, then realized that he had to finish what he had started. So, he stopped, and the rest of the poop came out.

Got me thinking...

Our world is full of so many distractions these days.

I realized that distractions had become my comfort zone. My phone, games, social media, TV, and even sports.

It is so easy to just get out the phone, play that game, check the social media, or check the email. It is so easy to turn the TV on and watch nothing. Is the smartwatch pinging you with every text message or notification?

There are other things that are more important. Like Duder, you need to finish that poop. Don't let the distractions control you.

At some point, you have to make a choice. What is more important to you? The sooner you make that choice, the better off you will be.

DUDER IS ALWAYS CURIOUS

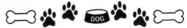

When I would take the pups out for a hike or a run, one of their more powerful senses is smell. They are constantly chasing down that scent. It may be off the trail, but they must follow and explore what they smell.

This can be good and bad. There have been a couple of times where I have seen them head off the trail to follow a smell. I see them stop and look at something, then I hear the rattle of the rattlesnake. Woah!! I have to start yelling at the dogs to leave that snake alone! Luckily, we have not had any major issues and they have never been bitten.

Even though it can be a bit dangerous, seeking out new things and wanting to see what is out there is a good thing.

Got me thinking...

I needed to do something different in my life. One of the biggest impacts was to begin learning again. It started by listening to podcasts instead of music and reading books instead of watching TV. I had to deliberately incorporate the process of learning into my life to the point where I wanted to continue learning everything I could.

This is a great example of the inputs we put into our minds. The more ideas and knowledge you put in, the more you can generate yourself. Every piece of information I've had come into my mind has had an impact of some sort. It all plays a role in how I think and view the world. I have gone back and listened to a podcast for a second time and have gotten something different out of it than the first time around.

Make this a habit. Stay curious and always learn.

SIMPLE GESTURES

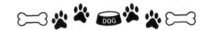

When Duder and I hop into the truck and head out for our hike, he rides in the back seat and waits for us to reach our destination. Sometimes he will reach up and put his head on my shoulder—maybe because he's feeling anxious, or maybe it's because I am. I love it when he does this. It is a very affectionate gesture, and he seems to always do it during the moments I need it the most. How does he know? What is it about dogs that they know when you need them? It's like they know how you're feeling and will respond to help you in any way that they can.

There are some cool things that dogs can do to assist their owners, which is why there are so many emotional support dogs and service animals. But it doesn't take extensive training for dogs to help out; sometimes it is the simple gestures, like Duder putting his head on my shoulder, that are enough.

Got me thinking...

I began experimenting with this idea. I started doing simple gestures towards the Blonde. Look her in the eyes and smile. Hold her hand in unexpected moments. Give her little back massages. I do these things in hopes that they will make her feel even a little bit better, and they will always be worth it.

DUDER'S CHALLENGE

What are some small things and simple gestures that you can do for the people around you? How can you improve the day of your kids, your coworkers, and even strangers? How can you have a positive impact on people?

Start making a conscious effort to be kind to those around you. Even offering someone a smile and a greeting counts; it's so much better than giving them a look that practically screams, "Leave me alone!"

Remember that no act of kindness is too small. People take what others give them and pass it on, whether it's positive or negative, so try to leave positive impressions on people so they can feel good as well.

FOOTPRINTS WE LEAVE

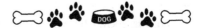

Duder and I were out for a hike, and there was some very soft dirt both on the trail and in tall hills. Duder was running all over the place, climbing the hills of dirt and leaving his footprints everywhere he went.

Got me thinking....

We are leaving "footprints" all the time.

Everywhere we go, either on foot, in the car, or on the plane, we have an impact. Every person we encounter impacts us, an vice versa. Everything we do in our community has an impact. With every interaction with our families, we have an impact.

These are the footprints we leave.

On the trails, when Duder and I are backpacking or hiking, we follow the basic rule of, "If you pack it in, you pack it out."

I am passionate about taking care of the trails and mountains. They have given a lot to me, and I try to give back to them. On some hikes, I will take time to do some basic maintenance. This might include clearing out debris, fixing spots where erosion has happened, and picking up other people's garbage. The trails are a place where I like to go, and I want to do my part to take care of them.

This thinking has allowed me to pay closer attention to all of my footprints. This includes the impact on the environment and our planet. It also includes impact on my community. What should I be doing to assist my neighbors, my city, my church, and my schools? I consider it all now.

Sometimes the footprints we leave are the steps we do not take. I took some serious reflection on this idea. Are there other things I should be doing? Are there things I could be doing, but am not?

DUDER'S CHALLENGE

Take some time to evaluate the footprints you are leaving in the world. How do you impact the world, your community, and even your home? Do your footprints need to change?

DUDER LOVES STAR TREK

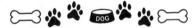

Duder has a doggy bed that is shaped like Captain Kirk's chair. Duder and I have a *Star Trek* headboard. He will sometimes sleep on a *Star Trek* blanket. He even has a *Star Trek* name tag. With all this stuff, he must love *Star Trek* right? Okay, maybe he doesn't, but I have always been a fan.

As a *Star Trek* fan, one thing I have always wanted to do was go to a *Star Trek* convention. In my new state of mind, I decided that now was the time. I found an upcoming show in Las Vegas, signed up, and decided to ride my motorcycle down. I planned out my route, what I was going to wear, where I would stay, and what events at the show I wanted to attend. I should mention that I ride a Kawasaki Vulcan 900 classic. I should also mention that my clothing of choice was a Spock outfit. (For you non-trekkies, Spock is a Vulcan.) I was cruising down the Las Vegas Strip on my motorcycle and in my Spock outfit. I was a Vulcan on a Vulcan, going to hang out with some other Vulcans.

Got me thinking...

I talk a lot in this book about doing things differently, discipline, and future-self concepts. But life is what you make it, and it isn't all about controlling yourself and living a strict life. I want to be happy, too. Doing things like riding my motorcycle and checking off a bucket list item like a *Star Trek* convention are things that make me happy.

No matter your age in life, find the things that bring you joy and long-term happiness—and notice that I said "long-term" and not "short-term" happiness. It would be easy to use this idea as an excuse or rationalization to do things that are gratifying in the present moment. There are plenty of things that don't benefit you in the long run and only bring very short-term rewards. I had to find the balance and recognize the things that I thought made me happy in the past, but were only hurting me.

CHASING SHADOWS

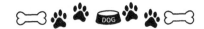

Duder is obsessed with light and shadows. If you shine a laser, Duder, like most dogs, will go nuts. Sometimes we will be in our family room and the light coming through the window will cast a small shadow on the wall. Duder will get on the couch and just stare or paw at it. I have seen him sit there and stare at it for more than thirty minutes. He is obsessed and can't stop worrying about it.

Got me thinking...

What are the shadows in my mind? We all have them. Some of them might be small events that, for some strange reason, get stuck in there. Some of them might be traumatic events. Either way, these shadows can haunt us and pull us out of our current reality and back into the past.

I have a few shadows—nothing that seems too traumatic on the surface, but occasionally, they'll pop into my mind and won't go away. They will overtake my current thoughts and feelings. I can be with people or by myself, and these shadows will affect my emotions and my state of mind. Sometimes, Duder will notice something is up, that I am feeling a little down, and he will casually walk over to say hello to me.

When the shadows from your past resurface, sometimes all you need is something in the present to ground you. For me, it's Duder coming to check on me. These moments can be great, because they pull my focus away from the shadows and onto something that brings light to my life.

DUDER GOT NEUTERED

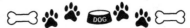

As Duder was getting older, the idea of getting him neutered came up. When we started researching the process, it hit me hard that they essentially chop his balls off. When I read that, I did the normal guy thing: cringed a bit and covered my own private area as a protective measure. Remove his balls? Woah. I felt bad for him. You never want to do that to a guy.

But we went through the procedure, we felt it was necessary for him. After the procedure, one of my daughters asked me, "Dad, are you going to make a Duder blog post about losing your balls? You guys have so much in common!"

Got me thinking...

Though I haven't been neutered, I have had a vasectomy, which is what I consider to be the humane human version of being neutered. My procedure experience was a little different than Duder's. They put him to sleep to do the chopping, but they did not put me to sleep.

I made the mistake of letting the Blonde come with me to the procedure. (Guys, I'm telling you now: DON'T do this.) I even let her come into the room where the event took place. Here's how it went down. The nurse tells me to strip down and lay on the operating table as she begins prepping me. The doctor comes in with a smile, a scalpel, and a whole slew of vasectomy jokes. At this point, the Blonde is sitting in the corner and trying to stifle a giggle. This giggling is contagious, and the nurse and doctor both start giggling as well. I am lying on this frickin table, fully exposed, with people working on my privates, and all parties involved are laughing away.

Maybe they should have just put me to sleep and chopped my balls off.

MAKING THE BLONDE HAPPY

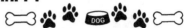

If anyone follows @duderandroxie on Instagram, you know that the Blonde loves to dress the dogs up. Sometimes I feel bad for them. I mean, come on, dogs aren't supposed to be dressed up like that! It's pure torture, right? I see all the work that the Blonde goes through to get them to sit still while she puts clothes on them, then to make them sit still while she takes all the pictures.

So, why do the dogs go through all that? In their case, they get rewarded with treats and attention.

Got me thinking...

Does the Blonde want me to do things that I don't want to do? Of course. When I think about it, I am no different than Duder. She wants to dress me up and pose for pictures the same way he does! I was wearing a plaid shirt the other day, and her first reaction was that it was a good color to match Duder. She called it the color of Duder. She dresses me to match Duder.

So, why do I go through all that? Because I get rewarded as well. It makes the Blonde happy, which in turn, makes me happy. That is my reward.

Why do we do anything in life? Do we always expect to get rewarded? Do we only do things if we get something in return?

How about service or charitable work for our fellow humans—do we only do this if we get something out of it?

Let's change the mindset a bit. We do it, and should do it, purely because we care. Purely because we should. I believe we are all born with a basic goodness in our hearts and want to help others because it is the right thing to do.

DUDER'S CHALLENGE

Go find a neighbor, family member, friend, or colleague that needs your time, help, or attention. Check in with them, ask if they need anything from you or if they'd like help with anything. Don't look for anything in return; just do it because you should.

INNER BEAST

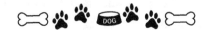

I take Duder and Roxie out for a hike or a run pretty much every day. Roxie will sometimes go into "beast mode" and focus in on Duder. She will attack him by trying to bite his collar, oblivious to anything else around her. Every ounce of her attention is on him.

Sometimes, the two of them will see a rabbit or a squirrel, and they switch to beast mode and chase that rabbit right up the side of a mountain at full speed. They have never actually caught one, but that does not stop them from trying.

Got me thinking...

As I was losing weight and began more intense exercising, running became my exercise of choice. When you start out, running is hard. Very hard. You do eventually reach a point where running is no longer a chore.

One of the ways I kept myself motivated was to sign up for races. Once you have that race on the calendar, you know you must train and get your miles in so you will be ready.

In my training, I would sometimes pretend I was chasing that rabbit. I would call on my inner beast to keep running. There were times when I would hit a wall and wanted to stop, when I could not run anymore, but that rabbit was still out there. I still had to chase it. I still had something inside of me that needed to catch it. That rabbit was always in front, and I had to keep running.

In northern Utah, running during the winter can be a challenge. It is cold, snowy, and icy. Early in my running journey, I wrote some affirmations on my whiteboard. One of them was: "I am a runner." This is a bold and very definitive statement for who I am. I use this statement as a "kick in the ass statement" to get me out the door. I am an early morning runner. There have been times when it is 5:00 a.m. and around 10°F outside. Those are the times when it is the most difficult to walk out the door. Those are the moments that truly define us.

I would set my intentions that night before and have a plan. I would lay out all my gear, decide how long to run, and plant the basic mindset to what needed to be done. I would go to bed with the intention and anticipation of running the next morning.

Make your statements of who you are. Write them down. Then the actions required to be that person will come easier.

LEARNING TO LIVE TOGETHER

When Daisy came along, and then Roxie, there were times of strife with Duder. The dogs had to figure out how they were going to get along, and they needed to figure out the answers to some basic questions. Who is the boss? Who eats first? Who goes out the door first? Where do I pee and poop? Where do I sit and sleep?

Over time, they learned how to get along. They got closer, and learned each other's patterns. They each had their own personalities.

Got me thinking...

The Blonde and I have been married for over thirty-seven years. We were eighteen when we were married, and we are now in our mid-fifties. That is a lot of time to learn from each other.

I do not have a secret to marriage or relationships. A relationship is two unique individuals trying to live a life together, so there's no end all be all rule to follow to have a successful relationship. While going through my transformation, though, I learned and focused on a few different things that helped me.

- There is more than one side to every relationship, but the truth is that you can only control your side of things. Own your decisions, and take accountability for all of your actions and reactions. Placing blame on someone for a problem that both of you have to deal with isn't going to help. The cause of a problem is irrelevant; what matters is your response to the issue and how you plan to resolve it.

- The reason the Blonde and I are still together is because we both choose to be. Every day, we must consciously choose to be to be together and to stay together.

- Having some bumps in the road is natural. Just like a trail run is varied and all over the place, our relationship is bound to have some rocky patches and ups and downs. It's all part of the journey, and really, these winding roads help keep things interesting.

- Intimacy is important. Everyone has different needs, and we each respond to sex differently. Each person within the relationship should clearly express what their needs are, and their partner should do what they can to meet these needs. The Blonde and I had some dry spells in our sex life, and it was mostly because of my laziness and lack of physical health. When I lost weight got my body operating properly, the sex and intimacy became much, much better.

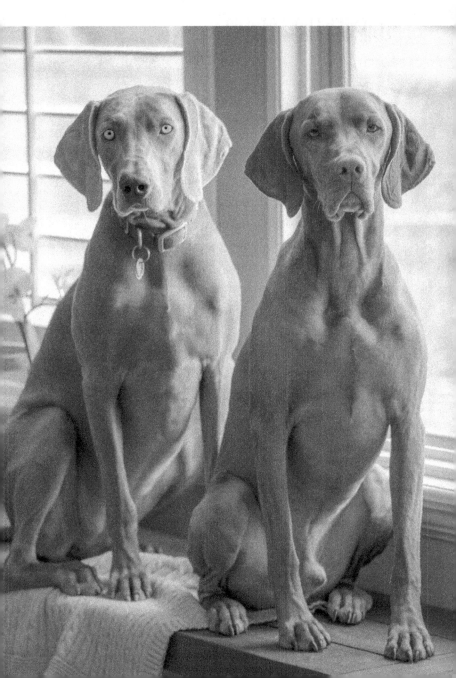

LEARNING FROM OTHERS

When I take Duder and Roxie out for a hike, sometimes Duder will get into full hunting mode. He must hear or see something, but he stops and gets into his pointing stance, just like a good pointer should do. I was watching this one day and noticed that as soon as Duder did this, Roxie did as well. She was not close to Duder and did not see the same thing as Duder; she was simply responding to him. Her instincts took over. She was learning and duplicating what Duder was doing. Maybe she didn't even know why. This is pure instinct, referred to as the "prey drive," and is very prevalent in our two breeds.

Got me thinking...

Who do we follow and learn from? Who are our mentors? Who inspires us?

During my transformation, I have had to rethink this idea. I started to ask myself who I was trying to be like. Who were the ones that I looked up to? Who inspired me?

I am not going to spend time talking about who inspires me—there are many. But what I will say, as I get older, this list gets smaller and closer to me. It is not about celebrities or famous athletes anymore. I get so much more inspiration from my four-year-old granddaughter. There's so much to learn from her simple wisdom and wondrous view of the world. She is unfazed and provides me with plain and pure happiness. In many ways, I am like a four-year-old again myself. A new world has opened up for me, and I am exploring it with my eyes wide and in wonder.

I also have a much better appreciation for everything I can learn from the Blonde, my kids, and all my grandkids. All of them are in different stages of life. There is so much to learn from all of them and their perspectives on things. These are my true mentors.

If you need to learn from someone, you may find that the best teachers are with you already.

ARE DOGS BETTER THEN KIDS?

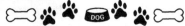

"You can stand in the light. And you can set a positive example. But you simply cannot make someone change." —Rich Roll

The Blonde and I have three daughters and four grandkids (three granddaughters and one grandson). Raising kids can be hard. It can be challenging, heartbreaking, and frustrating.

Dogs, on the other hand, can be all those things, but at least you can train them to behave. They will learn to obey you, and they will even do their chores.

Kids are a different story. It is hard to train your kids; they will resist, and ice cream can only go so far to sway them.

Got me thinking...

I have fully embraced this notion that kids have to find their own way in the world. I had to find my own way.

My role as a parent was to teach them what they might need to know to make their own choices and decisions in the world, not to always make those choices for them. They might fail throughout their lives, and they might get embarrassed because of one of their choices. They might even hate me sometimes, but I always wanted them to be equipped to handle anything and everything that may come their way.

What I have realized is that one of the best methods I can do to influence my kids is to do what I say I will do—which is to say, I show them the integrity of my character. I want to set an example for them through my actions, and I want my actions to reflect my words.

I had what I call a "father moment" the other day. My middle daughter has taken up running like I have. She has set a goal to run fifty half marathons—one in each of the fifty states. That is a frickin awesome goal! She recently bought herself some new running shoes, and of course, she had to share a pic of them with me. The Blonde and I were in the car, and we called her to talk about her new shoes. She said they are going work well for her; they've already reduced some of her hip pains. She then described that the sales guy helping her at the running store was asking her why she runs. My daughter told him that she runs because of her dad. Her dad lost weight and now runs marathons and ultramarathons.

Boom. I could not talk. The tears were coming down. This father moment was awesome. She runs because I inspired her with my running. These moments are what being a dad is all about.

She also finished her first marathon in October of 2022. She was able to run the Marine Corp Marathon, running through downtown Washington, D.C. I'm very proud of her.

Side Note: My youngest daughter also ran a marathon about four years ago, so two of my kids have run a marathon. I still need to work on that third one.

My actions and examples are influencing my kids. The best thing I can do as a dad is by doing things that might inspire them to keep moving forward.

SCIENCE OF DOGS

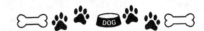

There have been numerous studies that highlight the power and the science behind how a dog can impact someone's life.

Some of the specific results that come from the studies include:

- Dogs can genuinely make us happier.
- They alleviate stress and anxiety and make us feel less alone.
- They keep us moving.
- They make us love them, which encourages our love of others.
- Having a dog as a pet improves our cognitive functions.

Basically, simply having a dog in your life has influence over you. Small and subtle lessons, habits, feelings, and influences will embed themselves into your life.

The Blonde and I have both experienced the healing power of dogs in our lives. Duder saved my life by opening my mind to possibilities and pushing me to explore them

DUDER IS ALWAYS THERE FOR ME

If I am ever feeling down, stressed, or a little sad, all I have to do is call Duder's name. He will always come running to me with his tail wagging and a smile on his face.

I can always count on him to be there for me. He always brings me back to simplicity.

Life is as complicated as we make it for ourselves, and Duder reminds me that things don't have to be complicated. Simple things can make all the difference.

DUDER WILL NOT BE HERE FOREVER

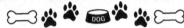

Dogs do not live as long as humans. It is very likely that Duder will pass on before me. This is a topic that I have chosen to not to think about very often. I don't want to lose my best friend.

Got me thinking...

Duder's influence got me this far in my transformation journey. He continues to inspire me and keep me moving forward every day. He is a core part of my "why" that gets me up every day, and he provides me with a sense of excitement for what I do.

It will be a very sad day when Duder is no longer with us, because his impact has spanned further than just the time he's been in my life. He saved me, transformed my future, and pushed me to reflect on my past in order to make something out of it.

He has had such a big influence on me, so what am I going to do when he is gone? Am I going to be able to keep going? How will I stay motivated?

As you have read in this book, there are many ideas and concepts to incorporate into your life. As I have processed these ideas and lived them, the idea of "lifestyle" keeps coming up. I need to stay on the path and continue to do things I have started. This is the lifestyle that I have chosen, and it's how I plan to continue to live.

What I do is no longer a collection of daily choices I am making. I am not doing these things until I reach some goal. I am no longer dependent on Duder to inspire and motivate me. It is my lifestyle. It is who I am.

But having a Duder Jr. wouldn't hurt...

LIFE IS A TRAIL RUN

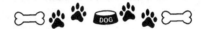

There is no end to this trail. There is no stopping point. It goes on and on and on.

There are hills to climb, rocks to navigate, and twists, turns, and hazards to watch out for along the way.

There are also easy sections: downhill, smooth, and straight.

You are always with yourself on the trail. You might have a partner or companion on the trail with you as well—maybe even a couple of dogs. You are all in it together.

There is beauty all around. There are trees, rocks, dirt, flowers, rivers, and waterfalls. There's a great deal to absorb and appreciate, so let the sun warm you, breathe the clean air, listen to the sounds surrounding you, and smile.

Life truly is about the journey.

AN AFTERWORD FROM THE BLONDE

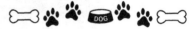

Jeff and I got married at a very young age. I was eighteen and pregnant, and marriage felt like the only option for us. We tried—we really did—but of course, we were young and immature. Resentment was easier to grow than friendship. We went through it: school, work, moving, his epilepsy. We went through so many trials, and years later, we found ourselves with three children and not a lot of love for each other. I played victim and he played dead. The blame game was our go-to, and we were unhappy.

As the years went by, I grew to be slightly neurotic, while Jeff seemed to become entirely apathetic. He didn't care about his body or health, he had terrible hygiene, and there was a permanent imprint on the couch from his bum. I was often walking on eggshells around him, not knowing if he was going to be a cranky-ass that day, and he had to do the same for me. We were both so irritable, even when there was no reason for it.

Trying to fix our relationship or asking him for anything often resulted in yelling matches. We would fight over nothing, and neither of us were going about resolving things in the correct way. I was miserable, not sleeping, and on too much medication. I was planning on leaving him.

Then we decided to get Duder.

Duder was the cutest little rambunctious puppy. He was the chubbiest pup in the litter, he loved food, and he shared Jeff's birthday. We took it as a sign—it was kismet.

Vizsla's need a lot of exercise, and that was Jeff's job. He started walking Duder every day, then they started running. He went on Keto and lost weight. He started to care! At first, I was jealous of Duder. Jeff let his dog sleep in the same bed as him, and he showed so much love for Duder. But I later realized that Jeff's shortcomings had nothing to do with me, and whatever motivation he could find to seek happiness was what he needed to work for. Plus, he snores, and I need my sleep.

Now he is on a quest for growth and improvement for his mind and body. He wants to take care of himself so we can have a quality life together. I am so proud of him for getting off the couch and running marathons. He has raised his vibration, and his energy is so much better. His attitude took a complete 180, he has a zest for life, and we are both finally trying to find our own happiness. We stopped trying to fix each other and started focusing on fixing ourselves, and that is what brought us closer together. I'm glad I didn't leave him, and I'm excited for our future together.

—The Blonde

APPENDIX

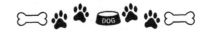

I have seen the "power" of dogs to heal and comfort. I know how dogs have influence and have an impact on people's lives.

To give you an idea of some of the organizations out there that bring dogs and people in need together, this is a short list of organizations that provide services for both people and dogs.

Labs for Liberty

https://www.labsforliberty.org/

Our mission is to acknowledge, honor, and empower members of United States Special Operations Forces by providing service dogs for PTSD and physical needs.

No one goes to war and returns unchanged. Some of our warriors return home uncertain as to their true identity. Labs for Liberty's goal is to support veteran's needs to overcome wounds of the past and enjoy life in a new light.

Pets for Vets

www.petsforvets.com

A Bridge to a Better Life

Many brave troops return home with scars – both seen and unseen – that make it difficult to transition back to civilian life. At the same time, millions of wonderful animals wait in shelters for a forever home. Pets for Vets is the bridge that brings them together.

When a Veteran is matched with the right pet, both lives change for the better. The Veteran saves the animal and welcomes him/her into a loving home. The pet provides the Veteran with unconditional love and support, easing stress, depression, loneliness and anxiety. Together, they share a Super Bond® that provides them both with a whole new "leash" on life.

PAVE - Paws Assisting Veterans

https://www.paveusa.org/service-dogs-for-veterans/

Service Dogs For Veterans

We provide custom-trained service dogs for Veterans free of charge with lifetime support.

While military service only lasts for a limited time,

the psychological and physical wounds experienced by Veterans can last forever. The healing process is a unique journey for every Veteran, and for some, every day is a challenge. From the roughly 2.7 million Americans that have deployed to Iraq and Afghanistan since 2001, it's estimated that 1 in 5 is experiencing Post Traumatic Stress Disorder (PTSD). Conditions like PTSD, MST, and TBI present numerous symptoms that disrupt daily living and make it difficult to sleep, socialize, and maintain independence.

Service dogs provide immense support for Veterans to improve their quality of life. Our purpose at PAVE is to help more Veterans access the benefits of service dogs. By offering customized training and lifetime support, we make a tangible and significant difference in the lives of Veterans.

Pets for Patriots

https://www.petsforpatriots.org/

Serving veterans and saving pets since 2010

Our work uplifts the lives of military veterans and their families while saving the most overlooked shelter dogs and cats

Guide Dogs of America
https://www.guidedogsofamerica.org/

Guide Dogs for people who are blind/visually impaired become trusted companions that bring new opportunities for life experiences and social interaction, as well as greater confidence and independence.

These highly trained canines help our clients travel safely from one destination to the next, avoiding obstacles, stopping at elevation changes, and looking out for all oncoming traffic, and remembering common routes.

Finding the right partner, forming a strong bond, and maintaining a solid support system are the keys to a successful guide dog partnership.

Pet Partners

https://petpartners.org/

At Pet Partners, we believe that the human-animal bond is a mutually beneficial relationship that improves the physical, social, and emotional lives of those we serve. We are motivated by connection, compassion, and a commitment to sharing this meaningful bond with everyone who can benefit from time spent with an animal.

Pet Partners is the national leader in demonstrating

and promoting the health and wellness benefits of animal-assisted therapy, activities, and education. With thousands of registered teams making more than three million visits annually, Pet Partners serves as the nation's most diverse and respected nonprofit registering handlers of multiple species as volunteer teams. Pet Partners teams visit in a wide variety of settings and in various communities across the country and beyond with patients in recovery, people with intellectual disabilities, seniors living with Alzheimer's, students, veterans with PTSD, people who have experienced crisis events, and those approaching end of life.

You can find Dude at dudeandduder.com

Printed in the USA
CPSIA information can be obtained
at www.ICGtesting.com
JSHW021513091023
49904JS00009B/58